WALKING QUEENS

D1569604

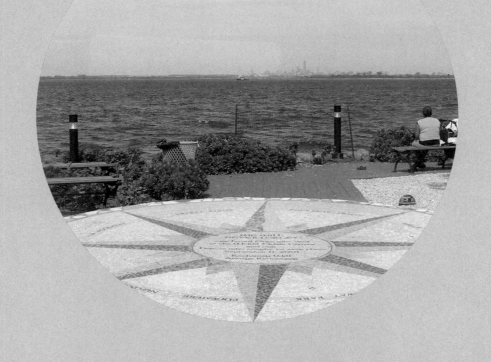

WALKING QUEENS

30 tours for discovering the diverse communities,
historic places, and natural treasures of
New York City's largest borough

Adrienne Onofri

 WILDERNESS PRESS ... *on the trail since 1967*

Walking Queens: 30 tours for discovering the diverse communities, historic places, and natural treasures of New York City's largest borough

First edition, first printing

Copyright © 2014 by Adrienne Onofri

Project editor: Ritchey Halphen
Editors: Laura Shauger and Amber Kaye Henderson
Cover and interior photos: Copyright © 2014 by Adrienne Onofri
Cartographer: Scott McGrew
Cover and book design: Larry B. Van Dyke and Lisa Pletka; typesetting and layout: Annie Long

Library of Congress Cataloging-in-Publication Data

Onofri, Adrienne.
  Walking Queens : 30 tours for discovering the diverse communities, historic places, and natural treasures of New York city's largest borough / Adrienne Onofri.
     pages cm — (Walking)
  Includes bibliographical references and index.
  ISBN 978-0-89997-730-0 (paperback) — ISBN 0-89997-730-8 — eISBN 978-0-89997-731-7
  1. Queens (New York, N.Y.)—Tours. 2. Walking—New York (State)—New York—Guidebooks. 3. Queens (New York, N.Y.)—Guidebooks 4. New York (N.Y.)—Guidebooks. I. Title.
  F128.68.Q4O66 2014
  917.47'24304—dc23

2014028309

Manufactured in the United States of America

Published by: **WILDERNESS PRESS**
                 An imprint of Keen Communications, LLC
                 PO Box 43673
                 Birmingham, AL 35243
                 800-443-7227; fax 205-326-1012
                 info@wildernesspress.com

Visit **wildernesspress.com** for a complete listing of our books, and for ordering information.

Distributed by Publishers Group West

Cover photos: *Front, clockwise from bottom left:* Flushing's Ganesha Temple; Wat Buddhathai Thavornvanaram, the Thai Buddhist temple in Elmhurst; Transfiguration Church, Maspeth; the Unisphere in Flushing Meadows Corona Park; the Robert F. Kennedy (Triborough) Bridge; Arbor Close in Forest Hills; Oakland Lake. *Back, top to bottom:* Little Neck Bay and the Throgs Neck Bridge; the Jam Master Jay memorial mural on 205th St. in Hollis; King Manor, Jamaica.

Frontispiece: Tribute Park in Rockaway (see Walk 30, page 236)

SAFETY NOTICE: Although Wilderness Press and the author have made every attempt to ensure that the information in this book is accurate at press time, they are not responsible for any loss, damage, injury, or inconvenience that may occur to anyone while using this book. Always check local conditions, know your own limitations, and consult a map.

acKNOWLEDGMENTS

At more than 330 years of age, Queens is just starting to emerge as a bona fide visitor destination. But there are organizations and people who have been working for years, often on a volunteer basis, to preserve and promote its heritage and attractions. For their direct assistance with this book and/or their efforts in general on behalf of Queens, I would like to thank the Queens Historical Society, Queens Tourism Council/Queens Economic Development Corp., Queens Library and its Queens Memory Project, Jack Eichenbaum, Donato P. Daddario, Carl Ballenas, Aquinas Honor Society of the Immaculate Conception School, Bayside Historical Society, Greater Astoria Historical Society, Jackson Heights Beautification Group, Greater Ridgewood Historical Society, Sunnyside Shines, Rego-Forest Preservation Council, Douglaston and Little Neck Historical Society, Newtown Historical Society, Richmond Hill Historical Society, Woodhaven Cultural & Historical Society, and all the Queens bloggers.

To anyone whom I neglected to mention by name but who deserves to be included, my gratitude (and apologies) to you also. I thank Molly Merkle and Wilderness Press for entrusting me with this project, Ritchey Halphen for his excellent work shepherding it through editing and production, and my family and friends for their encouragement. And special thanks to Daniel for your love, support, and patience.

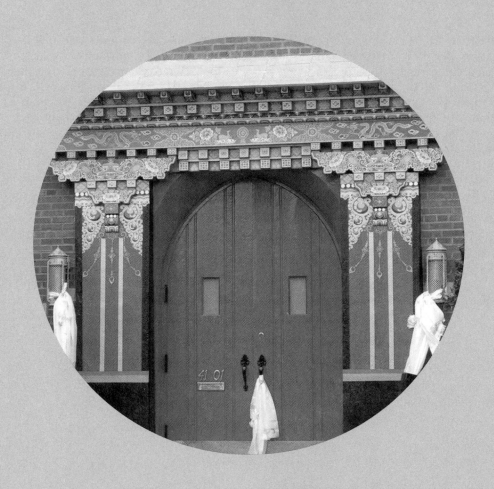

Doorway at the United Sherpa Association, formerly St. Matthew's Lutheran Church, in Elmhurst (see Walk 6)

AUTHOR'S NOTE

Traveling around Queens can be confusing. This is a laughable understatement to anyone who's ever done it, particularly without adequate preparation. You shouldn't have any trouble following the routes in this book: Each walk has a map and a step-by-step summary in addition to detailed directions. But a debriefing on the Queens street system would be helpful. Here goes . . .

The City of New York implemented a unified street grid in Queens: Numbered avenues run east–west; numbered streets run north–south. Problem is, most roads had been created within self-contained communities—old villages, planned developments, and so forth—so their length and orientation were not necessarily conducive to a boroughwide grid. As a result, no numbered street or avenue proceeds uninterrupted across Queens. Any one of them could get interrupted multiple times and disappear completely for a few blocks or even miles. Furthermore, some avenues are not on a straight east–west axis, and some streets are not due north–south; ditto for the boulevards (which have names). Plus, plenty of streets and avenues still have names, either because a neighborhood lobbied to keep them or for some other reason. And between any two avenues there may be a numbered road, drive, or terrace—or all three (for instance, going from 23rd Ave. to 24th Ave., you cross 23rd Rd., 23rd Dr., and 23rd Terr.); similarly, places and lanes are numbered with the streets. Other peculiarities exist as well.

You may find it helpful to bring along a Queens street map in case you decide to improvise after a walk, or you'd like to know where you are relative to the rest of Queens and how to get from one neighborhood to another. Be sure to have access to a Queens bus map (which also shows subway stops) in case you decide to explore further or need to curtail a walk. Maps are available at subway stations and on buses, or from the MTA website (**mta.info/nyct /maps/busqns.pdf**) or app (**mta.info/apps**).

Due to space limitations, we are unable to provide visiting hours for points of interest. Historic sites and art galleries may be open only a few days a week, or even just one day. Some points of interest on these walks are open seasonally. If you definitely want to go inside a particular place, check its hours in advance so you're sure to go on a day it's open. You may be able to arrange a visiting time outside of regular hours, as some historic houses will open by appointment.

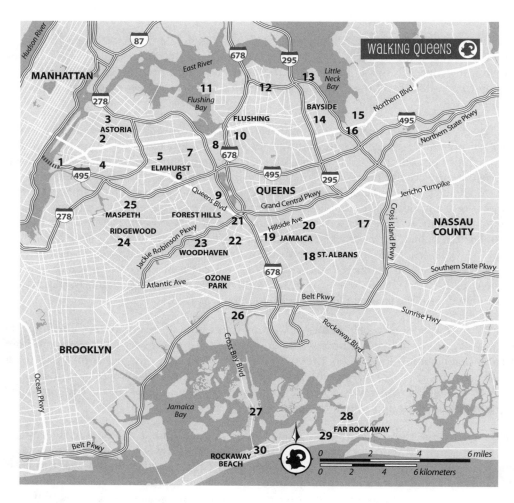

NUMBERS ON THIS LOCATOR MAP CORRESPOND TO WALK NUMBERS.

TaBLE OF CONTENTS

INTRODUCTION

While this book was being completed in 2014, the 50th anniversary of three significant events was commemorated. All three events—the Beatles' arrival in the United States, the Kitty Genovese murder, and the 1964 World's Fair—are known and had an impact internationally. And all three happened in Queens.

So why are people still under the impression that nothing, good or bad, ever happens in Queens? That it's just the place to put all those things Manhattan doesn't have room for— cemeteries, warehouses, car dealerships, airports? You even get that message from something that ostensibly celebrates Queens. In the final episode of the long-running sitcom *The King of Queens*, the title character, Doug Heffernan, and his wife go to China to adopt a baby. Holding his new daughter in his arms, Doug tells her: "You're gonna love Queens. Queens has got the New York Mets, it's got . . . well, not a lot else, actually."

No wonder Queens has been called the Rodney Dangerfield of boroughs! Dangerfield, by the way, is one of the many celebrities Queens has produced. It also produced a great American novel (*On the Road,* written by Jack Kerouac in his home on Cross Bay Blvd. in Ozone Park) and a great American document (the Flushing Remonstrance, which laid the groundwork for the Bill of Rights). UNICEF was established in Queens, where the UN General Assembly convened for its first five years. The world's first supermarket opened on Jamaica Ave. in Queens in 1930. Queens was the horse-racing capital of the United States for a time, the moviemaking capital at another. It's the birthplace of hip-hop (don't tell the Bronx), and where the greatest icons of jazz made their homes. All this, of course, is a mere sampling of its heritage.

Walking in Queens, you might observe a neighborhood's evolution in progress or discover centuries-old history. It could get you lost in the wilderness or set off your real estate envy. You'll see everything from factories to forts, contemporary-art galleries to classic architecture, storefront churches to elaborate temples. Home to more than 2.3 million people, with at least 150 different languages spoken among them, Queens has been heralded as the most multicultural place on Earth. The origins of its neighborhoods vary too: Some began as colonial villages, others as company towns, planned communities, summer resorts, or railroad suburbs. Queens also has diversity in nature—woodlands, glacial ponds, sandy ocean beaches, salt marshes, riverfront, meadows, and more. Take this book, slip into some comfortable shoes, and you're on your way to discovering all that Queens has to offer!

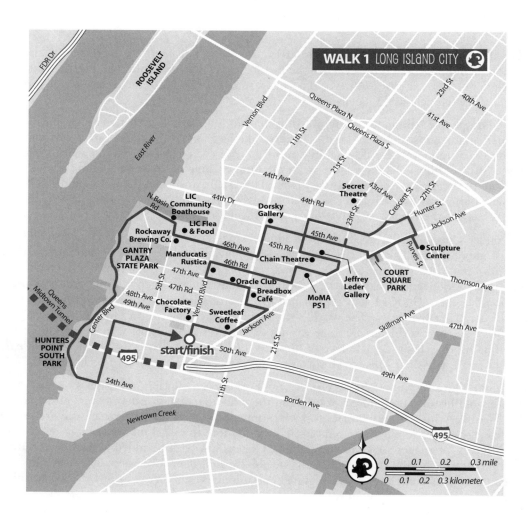

FDR Dr

ROOSEVELT ISLAND

East River

Queens Plaza N

Queens Plaza S

Vernon Blvd

11th St

21st St

23rd St

40th Ave

41st Ave

44th Ave

43rd Ave

Crescent St

27th St

Hunter St

Jackson Ave

Secret Theatre

44th Dr

44th Rd

N. Basin Rd

LIC Community Boathouse

Dorsky Gallery

45th Ave

LIC Flea & Food

Rockaway Brewing Co.

46th Ave

45th Rd

Sculpture Center

Purves St

GANTRY PLAZA STATE PARK

Manducatis Rustica

46th Rd

Chain Theatre

Jeffrey Leder Gallery

COURT SQUARE PARK

Thomson Ave

47th Ave

Oracle Club

5th St

47th Rd

Breadbox Café

MoMA PS1

Skillman Ave

47th Ave

Chocolate Factory

48th Ave

49th Ave

Vernon Blvd

Sweetleaf Coffee

Jackson Ave

Queens Midtown Tunnel

Center Blvd

start/finish

50th Ave

21st St

49th Ave

HUNTERS POINT SOUTH PARK

495

11th St

54th Ave

Borden Ave

Newtown Creek

495

0   0.1   0.2   0.3 mile

0   0.1   0.2   0.3 kilometer

LONG ISLAND CITY: RISING ON THE RIVER

BOUNDARIES: **43rd Ave., Jackson Ave., 54th Ave., East River**
DISTANCE: **4 miles**
SUBWAY: **7 to Vernon Blvd.–Jackson Ave.**

You see them from Manhattan, the Queensboro Bridge, and the 7 train: the glassy towers that have transformed Long Island City, or LIC, from a scruffy waterfront district shared by industry and artists to an ultraexpensive residential community whose views of—and convenience to—midtown Manhattan can't be beat. Most of the high-rises have been built since 2000, many of them since 2010. And more are coming, including two 40-plus-story condominiums slated to take the place of "graffiti mecca" 5Pointz, the enormous old warehouse that was covered in murals by artists from around the world and had been an unofficial landmark and tourist attraction. Once-independent Long Island City was incorporated in 1870 and accounted for a third of Queens' population when it was subsumed by New York City in the 1898 consolidation of what are now the five boroughs. Manufacturing has thrived there for more than a century and a half, and in just the past few years it has gotten a boost from the renaissance that has also elevated the cultural, retail, culinary, and office sectors.

- **Exit at 50th Ave. and Vernon Blvd., where you have a view of the Empire State Building. Walk in that direction on 50th Ave., but only as far as the 108th Precinct's station house on your right. This, *ahem,* arresting structure sports the city's seal rendered in stone, eagle sculptures at the windows, and an arched doorway flanked by columns and elaborately wrought lamps.**

- **Go back to Vernon Blvd. and make a left. Before the skyscrapers started rising, St. Mary's Church, at the next corner, had a hundred-year run as the only LIC building that could be seen from a distance.**

- **Turn right on 49th Ave. On your left as you reach Jackson Ave. is one of several 19th-century buildings in the neighborhood with fantastic terra-cotta ornamentation.**

- **Follow the building around to the left on Jackson Ave., where you can enjoy its historical interior along with a premium cup of coffee and fresh-baked treat at Sweetleaf.**

This spot where Jackson Ave. meets 11th St. is a very welcome one for runners in the New York City Marathon, as they've just passed the race's halfway mark by traversing the Pulaski Bridge from Brooklyn.

- Cross 11th St. to proceed on Jackson Ave. to the next large 1880s building showing off beautiful terra-cotta, at the corner of 47th Rd.

- Go left on 47th Rd., then right on 11th St. Breadbox Café, next to the gas station, is another place to get a baked good or beverage or sit down for a meal. The building was formerly an auto body shop; the restaurant owners created a new facade with 1,600 rolling pins engraved with the names of donors to Breadbox's charity partner.

- Turn left on 47th Ave. and proceed to the firehouse on the left. This 1903 Dutch Renaissance extravaganza resulted from the newly consolidated City of New York's efforts to upgrade the fire department's working conditions and public services. It was the only FDNY commission for Bradford Gilbert, the architect who'd given Manhattan its first skyscraper (the now-demolished Tower Building). Across the street, the library that you espy through the windows at #10-41 belongs to the Oracle Club, which artists and writers can join to gain access to work and social space, classes, and special events.

- Turn right on Vernon Blvd., Long Island City's "restaurant row," a 10-block stretch of acclaimed eateries ranging from burger joints to wine bars to places serving up fusion cuisine. Many of them have opened as the neighborhood has heated up, but Manducatis Rustica, on your right at #46-35, is run by a family that's been cooking old-country Italian for LIC for more than 35 years (this is their second location).

- Turn right on 46th Rd. Down the block on your right, a few old wood-frame houses bravely hold out in the midst of a condo intrusion. Their cute features, like bay windows and scalloped shingles, counterbalance the industrial nature of the other side of the street. Empire City Iron Works, across from the houses, is NYC's oldest steelmaker. Operating since 1904, the company has provided structural steel and ironwork for such legendary locales as the Metropolitan Opera and Yankee Stadium, as well as the new World Trade Center buildings.

● Walk one more block of 46th Rd. and turn left on 21st St. Before giving all your attention to the magnificent Romanesque home of MoMA PS1, check out the sign behind the flagpole on your left, which notes that this post office was named in honor of Geraldine Ferraro, the former Queens congresswoman, district attorney, and schoolteacher who ran for vice president on the Democratic ticket in 1984. The largest post office in 1920s New York, the building itself was honored with a listing on the National Register of Historic Places, with bronze doors, original lampposts, and roof balustrade among its standout details. Still, it's no match for the oldest public-school building in Queens across the street, with its great terra-cotta gables and finials, arch windows big and small, and variegated patterns in brick. Constructed in 1893 for children living in the 1st Ward of then-independent Long Island City (see the original school name above the door near 46th Rd.), it was renamed Public School 1 when Queens was incorporated into New York City. It was later rescued from abandonment by an artists' collective that evolved into the contemporary-art museum PS1, which added *MoMA* to its name when it became an affiliate of the Museum of Modern Art.

● Make a right on 46th Ave., looking at the old row houses on your left en route to the museum entrance at Jackson Ave. Ever since its first exhibition in 1976, PS1 (which has no permanent collection) has focused on site-specific art, putting the classroom configuration to use instead of remodeling it. Don't miss the old boiler room in the basement, where artists have covered the historical equipment in gold leaf.

● Turn left on Jackson Ave. and left again on 23rd St.

● Turn left on 45th Rd. On your right, mansard-roofed twin houses differentiated by paint jobs stand next to a Queen Anne town home with all kinds of flourishes from its bow window up—and its old address, 167, still on the door (it became 21-49 when street numbering was standardized boroughwide). Other nicely maintained circa-1890 homes are interspersed with commercial buildings and apartment houses on this mishmash of a street. Farther down, brownstones alternate with brick fronts in a graceful row that includes the Jeffrey Leder Gallery, featuring curated and juried art exhibitions in the town home at #21-37. Another cultural venue occupies the former U.S. Chain Co. building on your left, next to the white house: The Chain Theatre is part of Long Island City's off-Broadway scene (along with the Secret Theatre on 23rd St. and the Chocolate Factory on 49th Ave.).

- Make a right on 21st St.

- Turn right on 45th Ave., the neighborhood's showplace block from the time it was developed nearly 150 years ago right up to the present day. The first group of row houses on your right and most of the left side were designed by the same architects in the early 1870s and are united by an acanthus-leaf motif on the brackets below their rooflines. The first five houses on your right have a matched set on your left, the only two rows on the block faced in stone rather than brick. Note the stars on the brackets of the moldings over their first-floor windows. On the right, the single clapboard house dates to 1887, a few years older than the gabled trio next to it. The south side also has three tall 1889 apartment houses with distinctive brickwork between their bay windows.

  All the 1870–1890 homes on the block, including the apartment building at #21-48, compose the diminutive Hunters Point historic district. Hunters Point extends outside the landmarked area: It's considered a section of Long Island City (basically, west of the railroad tracks).

- Go left when you reach 23rd St., as the historic district extends around the corner to the row of five bowfront houses.

- Return to 45th Ave. Diagonally across the intersection from the landmarked houses is another attractive brick row. It's nice that all these lovely old houses survived the construction of an elevated train right on top of them, but isn't it crazy that an elevated train was constructed on top of lovely old houses?! Continue east on 45th Ave. until you're beneath the 50-story Citigroup Building at Jackson Ave. The green-hued office tower is the tallest building in New York City outside Manhattan (where it would rank about 55th) and the tallest on Long Island. While it now has high-rise company nearby, a skyscraper was an anomaly for Queens when the building opened in 1989.

- Cross to the south side of 45th Ave. and then to the other side of Jackson Ave., and go to your left. At the midblock entrance to Court Square Park, you have a picture-perfect view of the neighborhood's landmarked courthouse. It was built when the Queens County seat was relocated from Jamaica to Long Island City in 1870 and had to be rebuilt within the original walls after a fire gutted it in 1904. Two stories were added, two towers were eliminated, and all the exterior detail was replaced.

Of course, it's all that detail, including the ribbed metal roof, that makes it such an eye-catcher.

In a tawdry coda to the project, the architect, Peter M. Coco, was tried and convicted of extortion related to its construction, inside the very courthouse he designed. This is also the courthouse where Willie Sutton, standing trial in 1952, was asked by a journalist why he robbed banks and he replied, "Because that's where the money is." (The trial is fact, the quote possibly urban legend.) The two low wings flanking the courthouse, added in the 1930s, have sculptures of the blindfolded face of Lady Justice above their doors. Resume walking in the direction you had been going on Jackson Ave.

- Turn right at Purves St. to visit SculptureCenter, which produces exhibitions and related programming. Its building, on your left, was remodeled by Maya Lin—best known for designing the Vietnam Veterans Memorial in Washington, DC—when SculptureCenter moved here after more than 70 years in Manhattan.

- As almost all these short streets south of Jackson Ave. dead-end at railroad tracks, return to Jackson, cross the avenue, and head north on 43rd Ave. (which virtually aligns with Purves).

- Turn left on Hunter St., then fork right onto 44th Rd. as you approach the triangle. Small oases have been staked out amid all the new construction. The cute little park to your right resulted from the greening of an asphalt lot and is a placeholder for future constructioh. Across from it is a landscaped sitting area with a sundial and plaques paying tribute to

Row houses in the Hunters Point historic district

"everyday heroes," including Brian Watkins, the Utah tourist stabbed to death in the subway while visiting New York for the US Open in 1990.

- Walk toward the Citigroup Building and turn right on 44th Dr., between 1 and 2 Court Sq. Citigroup added #2 some 15 years after opening the tower at #1. When you reach 23rd St., look to your left at 1890s town houses that really deserve to be unobscured by an el. On the next block of 44th Dr., the union hall at #21-42 reveals its former owner in its entertaining ornamentation. The Benevolent and Protective Order of Elks abandoned this lodge in the 1920s for a now-landmarked building in Elmhurst that has a full elk (statue) out front.

    The Industry condominium across the street was the first local residential development by the owners of Silvercup Studios, one of LIC's best-known corporate residents, thanks to its huge rooftop sign. Silvercup has 13 soundstages in two buildings, where movies and such TV shows as *Girls, The Sopranos, Gossip Girl,* and *Sex and the City* have been filmed.

- Turn left on 21st St.

- Make a right on 45th Ave. At the end of the block, on your right, Dorsky Gallery promotes contemporary visual arts through publications, symposia, and exhibitions, which are curated independently (not by someone on staff) and often deal with current issues.

- Turn left on 11th St.

- Turn right on 46th Ave. It's just two blocks to 5th St., where the LIC Flea & Food outdoor market is open every weekend April–October. To your left at the 5th St. corner, you can have a beer drawn on tap at the very brewery where it's made. Rockaway Brewing Co. was started by a couple of guys who home-brewed in their Rockaway backyard, their specialty an English-style ale. Serving hours are 3–8 p.m. Thursday and Friday and noon–8 p.m. Saturday and Sunday.

- Go north on 5th St., walking with LIC Flea on your right. At the end of the street, turn left and walk alongside Anable Basin. If the time is right, step off the pavement and paddle a kayak into the East River: On most weekends when the flea market is open, the volunteer-run LIC Community Boathouse offers free kayak rentals.

● From the basin, begin your walk in Gantry Plaza State Park, which covers 12 riverfront acres encompassing piers, coves, playgrounds, lawns, and a fun variety of seating from which to enjoy these amazing views. Near the north end of the park, you walk right in front of the iconic Pepsi-Cola sign, erected when Pepsi opened a bottling plant in Long Island City in the 1930s. Pepsi shut down its LIC operations in the late 1990s, and the neon billboard is not only incorporated into the new residential development surrounding it but also partly inspired the development's design, as the building behind the sign was given curved edges to echo the swirls in the Pepsi lettering. (The 25- to 42-story buildings of this mega-development around the sign contain more than 2,600 apartments, plus gyms, children's playrooms, outdoor tennis courts, and a sandy volleyball court for residents.)

As you follow the riverside paths, you can stop to relax in a chaise longue, Adirondack chair, or high-backed seat tilted for your sunning convenience. Keep walking until you reach the park's namesake, the massive gantry cranes that used to transfer cargo between boat and train. You can still find some old rail tracks within the landscaping near the southern gantry.

● Continue south from Gantry Plaza via the path to Hunters Point South, a magnificently designed city park that opened in 2013. Located between 51st and 54th Aves., the park features a pavilion, a green oval, a (nonswimming) beach, and a wood-planked promenade with seating. You can board a ferry to Manhattan and Brooklyn from a terminal in the park. The nearest subway is at Vernon Blvd. and 50th Ave., about 0.4 mile away.

POINTS OF INTEREST

Sweetleaf Coffee & Espresso Bar sweetleaflic.com, 10-93 Jackson Ave., 917-832-6726

Breadbox Café breadboxcafelic.com, 47-11 11th St., 718-389-9700

The Oracle Club theoracleclub.com, 10-41 47th Ave., 917-519-2594

Manducatis Rustica manducatisrustica.com, 46-35 Vernon Blvd., 718-937-1312

MoMA PS1 ps1.org, 22-25 Jackson Ave., 718-784-2084

Jeffrey Leder Gallery jeffreyledergallery.com, 21-37 45th Rd., 212-924-8944

Chain Theatre chain-theatre.org, 21-28 45th Rd., 646-580-6003

Secret Theatre secrettheatre.com, 44-02 23rd St., 718-392-0722

Chocolate Factory chocolatefactorytheater.org, 5-49 49th Ave., 718-482-706

SculptureCenter sculpture-center.org, 44-19 Purves St., 718-361-1750

Dorsky Gallery dorsky.org, 11-03 45th Ave., 718-937-6317

LIC Flea & Food licflea.com, 5-25 46th Ave., 718-866-8089

Rockaway Brewing Co. rockawaybrewco.com, 46-01 5th St.

LIC Community Boathouse licboathouse.org, 5th St. and N. Basin Rd.

Gantry Plaza State Park Center Blvd. and 49th Ave., 718-786-6385

Hunters Point South Park Center Blvd. and Borden Ave.

route summary

1. Walk west on 50th Ave. and then back east. Turn north on Vernon Blvd. from 50th Ave.
2. Turn right on 49th Ave.
3. Turn left on Jackson Ave.
4. Turn left on 47th Rd.
5. Make a right on 11th St.
6. Make a left on 47th Ave.
7. Go right on Vernon Blvd.
8. Turn right on 46th Rd.
9. Make a left on 21st St.
10. Turn right on 46th Ave.
11. Turn left on Jackson Ave.
12. Turn left on 23rd St.
13. Turn left on 45th Rd.
14. Turn right on 21st St.
15. Make a right on 45th Ave.
16. Dip in and out of 23rd St. to your left, then resume going east on 45th Ave.

17. Make a left on Jackson Ave.
18. Go right on Purves St. to SculptureCenter, then return to Jackson Ave.
19. Cross Jackson and get on 43rd Ave.
20. Make a left on Hunter St.
21. Go right on 44th Rd.
22. Turn left on Crescent St.
23. Make a right on 44th Dr.
24. Turn left on 21st St.
25. Turn right on 45th Ave.
26. Turn left on 11th St.
27. Make a right on 46th Ave.
28. Turn right on 5th St.
29. Turn left on N. Basin Rd., then follow the path south through Gantry Plaza State Park.
30. Continue via park path to Hunters Point South.
31. Walk to Vernon Blvd. and 50th Ave. for subway.

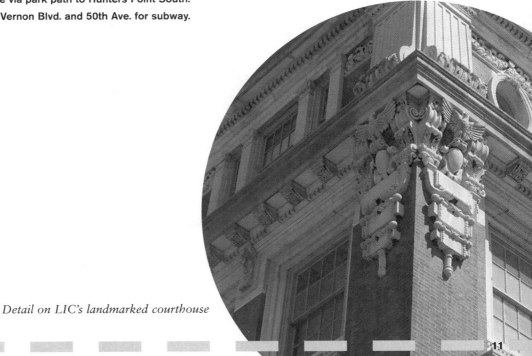

Detail on LIC's landmarked courthouse

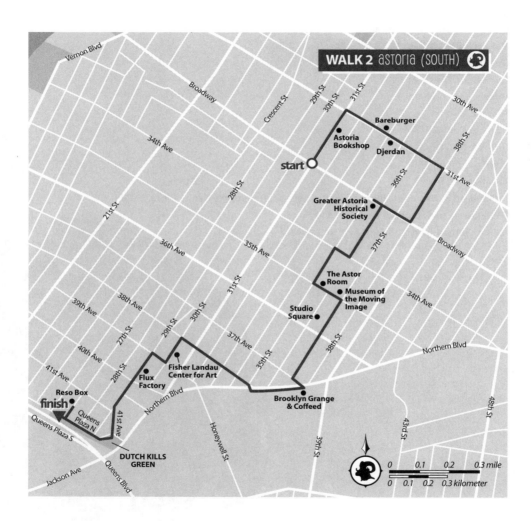

WALK 2 astoria (SOUTH)

Vernon Blvd
Broadway
Crescent St
29th St
30th St
31st St
30th Ave
38th St
31st Ave
34th Ave

Bareburger
Astoria
Bookshop
Djerdan
36th St

start

21st St
28th St

Greater Astoria
Historical
Society

37th St
Broadway

36th Ave
35th Ave
31st St

The Astor
Room
Museum of
the Moving
Image

34th Ave

39th Ave
38th Ave
36th Ave

Studio
Square

38th St

Northern Blvd

40th Ave
27th St
29th St
30th St
37th Ave
35th St

41st Ave
28th St

Fisher Landau
Center for Art

Flux
Factory

Reso Box
finish
Queens
Plaza N
Northern Blvd
41st Ave

Honeywell St

39th St

Brooklyn Grange
& Coffeed

48th St
43rd St

Queens Plaza S

**DUTCH KILLS
GREEN**

Jackson Ave
Queens Blvd

0   0.1   0.2   0.3 mile
0   0.1   0.2   0.3 kilometer

2 astoria (SOUTH): Grabbing THE SPOTLIGHT

BOUNDARIES: 31st Ave., 38th St., Queens Plaza, 27th St.
DISTANCE: 2.8 miles
SUBWAY: N or Q to Broadway

In 2000 *Time Out New York* wrote of Astoria, "Residents love the fact that their neighborhood is not, and probably never will be, trendy or gentrified." And that held true for another 10 years. Now, however, it's the coolest part of Queens. Whether it stems from a Williamsburg spillover or just a belated appreciation, Astoria has become the locus of buzz-generating developments in real estate, arts and culture, and dining. Its longstanding cultural institutions as well as newer art galleries are on this walk. You'll also pass by some trendsetting food and drink establishments, and you'll see how other players—from hoteliers to landscape designers—have been making an impact on this historic, multicultural neighborhood.

● Exit on the east side of 31st St. and cross Broadway to head north. The Astoria Bookshop at #31-29 is the only English-language, non-secondhand bookstore in western Queens, and the only independent bookstore in the whole borough.

● Turn right on 31st Ave. The house on your left at #31-07, built around 1875, is a lone survivor from when Jamaica Ave. (as 31st Ave. was then known) was a prestigious boulevard of mansions. Its exclusiveness waned with the construction of the elevated train in the 1910s. Across 33rd St., the Greek sign on the left marks the home of a fraternal organization for people from Lesbos. Also on this block is the original location of Bareburger, which has grown into an international chain of more than 20 restaurants in just five years. Its organic, all-natural menu includes not just the usual beef, turkey, and chicken burgers but also ostrich, elk, bison, and wild boar (and several vegetarian varieties). Another culinary mini-empire that started here is diagonally across the 34th St. intersection: Djerdan, which helped introduce New Yorkers to *burek,* a phyllo pie filled with meat, cheese, or spinach. On the next block, a club for fans of Athens's Panathinaikos soccer team shares a building at #35-07 with the Pythagoras Brotherhood, whose members hail from the Greek island of Samos. Representing an earlier population of Astoria is Trinity Lutheran Church, on your right as you near 37th St. It was founded by Germans in 1890 when they were Astoria's predominant ethnic group, and the congregation was still growing in the 1920s when this building was constructed. It's listed on the National Register of Historic Places, and its lovely interior features stained glass, woodwork, and a Skinner organ.

Past 37th St. on your left, Casa Galicia's building looks like it could have been built for this organization that celebrates Spanish heritage, but it originated as a catering hall in the 1920s.

● Turn right on 38th St. Among the ornamentation on homes on this block is 281 engraved within flora over the door of #31-82. That was the original building number—before the implementation of a Queens street grid.

● Turn right on Broadway. K&T Meats, on your right, played a key role in the Oscar-nominated movie *Julie & Julia:* It's where Amy Adams's character (who lives in Long Island City) shops when she decides to tackle Julia Child's beef bourguignonne recipe. The building on the left corner at 37th St. played a key role in, well, every office worker's life: Inside 32-05 37th St., a patent engineer named Chester Carlson invented the electrophotographic machine, which would become known as xerography. The first image Carlson reproduced was "10-22-38 ASTORIA," the date and place of his experiment; it took him until 1948 to find a buyer in Haloid, later rebranded Xerox.

Continuing down Broadway, you pass a Rite Aid building at 36th St. that must have been built for a Childs restaurant, as its polychromatic terra-cotta and roofline of seahorses were a hallmark of that defunct chain. Half a block away, fill in any gaps in your knowledge of the area at the Greater Astoria Historical Society, on the fourth floor of 35-20 Broadway. Their regular gallery hours are Monday, Wednesday, and Saturday afternoons, but they may open on request if you call or knock on the door. The society presents short- and long-term themed exhibits, as well as talks, panels, and performances. One important relic on permanent display is a door from Astoria's Blackwell mansion on which you can still see the arrow symbol British troops carved into property they seized during the American Revolution. The Blackwells were early settlers and major landowners in the area (Roosevelt Island, connected to Astoria by a bridge, was originally Blackwell's Island). In 1825, after the Blackwells had sold the home to Colonel George Gibbs, his friend James Fenimore Cooper came to visit and, according to some accounts, wrote his masterpiece *The Last of the Mohicans* during his stay.

Feelin' Groovy

In March 2011 the Queensboro Bridge was officially renamed the Ed Koch Queensboro Bridge. Just don't call it that around anyone from Queens. For them, it's the Queensboro Bridge and the Queensboro Bridge alone! Except, uh, when they call it the 59th Street bridge (for its Manhattan access point).

Former mayor Ed Koch—born in the Bronx, lived in Manhattan—had no personal or professional affiliation with Queens or the bridge. But people object to the renaming more because it shows such a lack of respect for Queens. The Brooklyn and Manhattan Bridges would never get co-named, would they? And no other bridge made such a difference for a borough as the Queensboro did. Opened in spring 1909, it was Queens' first vehicular link with Manhattan. Within 15 years, the population of Queens soared more than 250%, to 736,000. By 1930, it hit 1 million.

The Queensboro was the longest cantilever bridge in the world when it opened. Its tolls (starting at 3¢) were abolished in 1911. Originally, vehicles crossed on the lower level with trolleys; the upper deck carried pedestrians and trains. Today both levels are used entirely by vehicles, except for the pedestrian and bike lane on the north side of the lower level. The Queensboro Bridge carried the last trolley line to operate in New York City, until 1957.

F. Scott Fitzgerald wrote about the bridge in *The Great Gatsby.* Edward Hopper painted it. The opening credits of the 1970s sitcom *Taxi* track a cab driving across it. It's been prominently featured in such movies as *Spider-Man, Manhattan, City Slickers,* and *Nighthawks.* And the Simon and Garfunkel song better known by its subtitle "Feelin' Groovy" is named "The 59th Street Bridge Song."

- Go to 36th St. and make a right. You have a clear view to your left of the tower of Most Precious Blood, a Catholic church built in the 20th century with medieval influences. The small metal fence encircling the top of the tower is incised with peacocks. At 34th Ave., welcome to Hollywood East! Before this block was de-mapped in 2013 for the creation of the first outdoor soundstage in New York City, 36th St. was a through street. Kaufman Astoria Studios pays the city $140,000 annually to lease the block (the rent will increase every few years, naturally).

- Turn right on 34th Ave. and left on 35th St., walking beside the structure referred to in its landmark-designation report as Paramount Studios Building No. 1. It was erected for Famous Players Lasky Corp., which was cofounded by Cecil B. DeMille and Samuel Goldwyn, among others, and evolved into Paramount Pictures. It opened in 1921, and after more than 100 movies starring the likes of Rudolph Valentino, W. C. Fields, and Gloria Swanson had been filmed here, the studio closed briefly in 1927 to get equipped for production of talkies. After Paramount decamped for Southern California, the federal government acquired the studio. Most of the World War II propaganda films, including Frank Capra's Oscar-winning *Why We Fight* series, were made here. It continued to be used as the US Armed Forces' Signal Corps Pictorial Center until 1970.

- Make a left on 35th Ave., bringing you in front of Kaufman Astoria Studios, as it's been known since the early 1980s when it resumed regular commercial production under new owners. Expanded from one to seven soundstages, it's been the home of *Sesame Street* for more than two decades, and many movies and other TV series (including *Orange Is the New Black*) are shot here. The studio has served as the anchor of a burgeoning cultural corridor, formally designated the Kaufman Arts District by the city in 2014, that includes the Frank Sinatra School of the Arts across the avenue. This public high school was founded by Tony Bennett, born on 21st St. in Astoria, and named in honor of his friend and fellow music legend; the concert hall inside is named for Bennett. At 36th St., you see that not only does Kaufman Astoria now have a back lot like the LA studios, but it also has a large entry gate bearing the studio's name, à la Paramount's famous arch in Hollywood. In 2011 the old studio commissary was converted into a retro supper club named the Astor Room. Its entrance is behind the guard booth.

  Between 36th and 37th Sts., the Museum of the Moving Image's building was originally part of the studio complex. Visitors can create stop-motion animation, play video games, record film dialogue, and tinker with sound effects and music for well-known movies. The museum's permanent installations are a re-creation of a 1920s Egyptian-themed movie palace; the "Behind the Screen" exhibit, a comprehensive overview of the history, technique, and technology of filmmaking; and a retrospective on the work of Muppets mastermind Jim Henson scheduled to open in 2015.

● Turn right on 37th St. The brown lattice fence on your right encloses the outdoor lounge of Studio Square, inspired by the beer gardens that flourished in Astoria's German days (its entrance is on 36th St.).

● Turn left on 37th Ave. and continue a few yards to Northern Blvd. Across the boulevard is the Standard Motor Products building, which bends just like the road does. Standard manufactured auto parts in this 1919 building for some 75 years, but in 2008 it closed the factory and sold the building. It's still a tenant, as are a number of entertainment and media companies. The most impressive occupant, though, is Brooklyn Grange, a farm that takes up the entire roof. Produce is sold on-site when it's open to the public (Saturdays, spring–fall). The farm maintains a chicken coop and beehives, and it has some incredible views. Downstairs, Coffeed is also helping to develop this industrial area's environmental conscience. The café, which roasts its own coffee, is committed to eco-friendly practices in everything from sourcing beans to composting food waste.

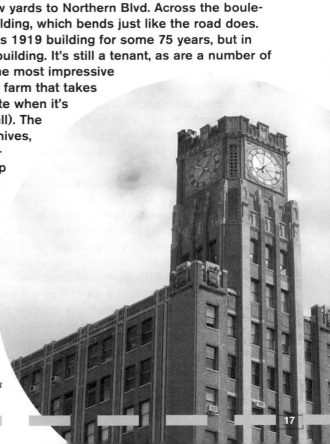

● With your back to the Standard building, go left on Northern Blvd.

● Cross 35th St. and fork right onto 38th Ave. Note the tires sculpted at the top of the building on your right,

The clock-tower building on Queens Plaza

#34-01. It was erected in 1913 as a service center for Pierce-Arrow, a luxury auto-mobile brand that ceased manufacturing during the Great Depression. The area from the Standard Motor Products building west to Queens Plaza was dubbed Detroit East in the early 20th century because of its many car-related businesses; Ford had both a plant and a dealership at Northern Blvd. and 31st St., and Rolls-Royces were assembled in a building at the end of this walk. Stay on the avenue past blocks of old frame houses and industrial sites, and under the elevated train.

● Turn left on 30th St. On your left toward the end of the block, the Fisher Landau Center for Art is a contemporary-art museum that grew out of a personal collection. Most of its exhibits feature selections from Emily Fisher Landau's trove of paintings, photographs, sculpture, prints, and other art from 1960 on, by such artists as Jasper Johns, Robert Rauschenberg, Kiki Smith, Cy Twombly, and Annie Leibovitz. The work is displayed on three airy, immaculate floors of a former parachute-harness factory.

● Turn right on 39th Ave., but not before noticing the elegant bay window of the corner house on your left, a Gilded Age town house onto which floors were recently added. Between 30th and 29th Sts., the whole left side is occupied by hotels, and there are also hotels to your right and around the corner—in fact, no fewer than 10 hotels are located within two blocks, almost all of them opened since 2010. This is the Dutch Kills section of Astoria—or, rather, Long Island City (you crossed into the LIC zip code around 37th Ave.). Europeans may have been farming at Dutch Kills, a tributary of Newtown Creek about a half mile south of here, as early as 1642, making it the very first European settlement in Queens. The original farmstead grew into a hamlet called Dutch Kills, which was merged with other villages (including Astoria) into the munici-pality of Long Island City in 1870.

● Make a left on 29th St. In the GREETING CARDS building on your left near the end of the block, Flux Factory supports and promotes emerging artists. Its exhibitions and interpretive events are typically collaborative projects focused on a physical, social, or cultural facet of NYC life. On this block, you also have a Catholic church, St. Patrick's, that's been around since the 1860s, and a Seventh-Day Adventist church started in the 1990s that is the only Filipino SDA congregation in the northeastern United States. On the next block, look above the door of the church to your left at its angel-adorned nameplate, and you'll see this was the First Reformed Church of Long Island

City, established in 1875. Newcomers High School, on the right, offers curriculum and services sensitive to the academic and social needs of immigrant students.

● Go left onto 41st Ave. and proceed across the next street into Dutch Kills Green, a park created in the $45 million refurbishment of Queens Plaza. The traffic-choked and clamorous corridor now has a greenway, culminating in this alfresco lunch spot for office workers. This park has also provided a home for two old millstones. Based on the sign here, it's been decided that they date from the 1800s and are not the ones from Burger Jorissen's 1650s mill—though some people contend they are, which would make them Queens' oldest European artifacts. Turn around to look at the clock tower, a 1927 office building erected for the Bank of Manhattan (see its monogram on the shields flanking the tower).

● Turn back and follow the blacktop path to your right through Dutch Kills Green to where it links up with the bicycle lanes, and cross Queens Plaza N. at 29th St. The huge building to your left was constructed in two phases, evident from the differing appearances of the lower (1917) and upper (1927) halves. Proceeding west, look around Queens Plaza to appreciate its multimillion-dollar revamp, which planted about 500 trees and small gardens, created biking and walking paths and sitting areas, and tremendously improved pedestrian crossings.

Between 28th and 27th Sts., JetBlue is headquartered in the 1911 Brewster Building, the first major structure to go up on the plaza after the Queensboro Bridge opened. You know the Cole Porter song "You're the Top," which name-drops all kinds of wonderful things? It used to have a lyric, which hasn't been sung in ages: "You're a Brewster body!" Those bodies—of Brewster cars—were manufactured here. The building later housed a Rolls-Royce of America assembly plant and, during World War II, airplane manufacturing.

● Make a right on 27th St. to visit Reso Box, a Japanese art gallery and café.

● The N, Q, and 7 station is on Queens Plaza at 27th St. Or go one more block and follow the pedestrian lane onto the Queensboro Bridge to walk to Manhattan—it's about a mile across.

POINTS OF INTEREST

Astoria Bookshop astoriabookshop.com, 31-29 31st St., 718-278-2665

Bareburger bareburger.com, 33-21 31st Ave., 718-777-7011

Djerdan djerdan.com, 34-04 31st Ave., 718-721-2694

Greater Astoria Historical Society astorialic.org, 35-20 Broadway, 718-278-0700

The Astor Room astorroom.com, 34-12 36th St., 718-255-1947

Museum of the Moving Image movingimage.us, 36-01 35th Ave., 718-777-6888

Studio Square studiosquarenyc.com, 35-33 36th St., 718-383-1001

Brooklyn Grange brooklyngrangefarm.com, 37-18 Northern Blvd., 347-670-3660

Coffeed coffeednyc.com, 37-18 Northern Blvd., 718-606-1299

Fisher Landau Center for Art flcart.org, 38-27 30th St., 718-937-0727

Flux Factory fluxfactory.org, 39-31 29th St., 347-669-1406

Dutch Kills Green Queens Plaza N. and 41st Ave.

Reso Box resobox.com, 41-26 27th St., 718-784-3680

route summary

1. Walk north on 31st St. from Broadway.
2. Turn right on 31st Ave.
3. Turn right on 38th St.
4. Make a right on Broadway.
5. From the Greater Astoria Historical Society, go east on Broadway.
6. Turn right on 36th St.
7. Make a right on 34th Ave.
8. Turn left on 35th St.
9. Turn left on 35th Ave.
10. Turn right on 37th St.
11. Turn left on 37th Ave.
12. Walk west on Northern Blvd.
13. Fork right on 38th Ave.
14. Make a left on 30th St.
15. Turn right on 39th Ave.
16. Turn left on 29th St.
17. Go left onto 41st Ave.
18. Make a right on Queens Plaza.
19. Turn right on 27th St., then return to Queens Plaza.

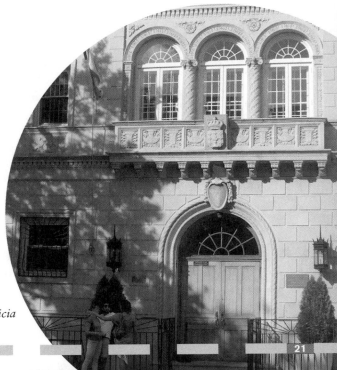

Casa Galicia

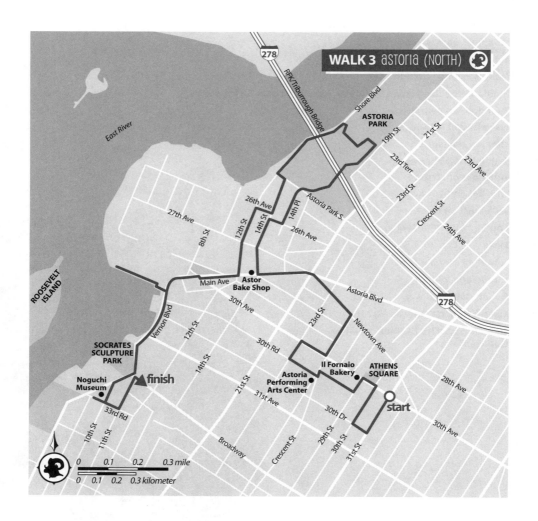

WALK 3 astoria (North)

278 RFK Triburrough Bridge

East River

Shore Blvd

ASTORIA PARK

19th St

21st St

23rd Terr

23rd St

23rd Ave

27th Ave

26th Ave

14th Pl

Astoria Park S

Crescent St

24th Ave

8th St

12th St

14th St

26th Ave

Main Ave

Astor Bake Shop

ROOSEVELT ISLAND

Vernon Blvd

30th Ave

Astoria Blvd

278

SOCRATES SCULPTURE PARK

12th St

14th St

30th Rd

23rd St

Newtown Ave

28th Ave

Noguchi Museum

finish

21st St

30th Ave

Astoria Performing Arts Center

Il Fornaio Bakery

ATHENS SQUARE

33rd Rd

31st Ave

start

10th St

11th St

Broadway

Crescent St

29th St

30th St

31st St

30th Dr

30th Ave

0   0.1   0.2   0.3 mile

0   0.1   0.2   0.3 kilometer

3 astoria (NortH): THe way THey were

BOUNDARIES: 23rd Terr., 31st St., 33rd Rd., Vernon Blvd.
DISTANCE: 4 miles
SUBWAY: N to 30th Ave.

Only Athens, it's been said, has more Greeks than Astoria. For many years, and to many people, that was Astoria's No. 1 identity, although *Mediterranean* would be more accurate because it's also had a lot of Italians and Croatians. Since the 1990s, Astoria has become more of a polyglot, with a significant influx of Bangladeshis, Egyptians, and Brazilians among other nationalities. Characterizing Astoria these days, however, you might bypass ethnicity altogether and refer to hipsters, artists, or some other term conjuring trendy and creative people. On this route, you will see the influence of the diverse populations who have called Astoria home over the years, going all the way back to founder Stephen Halsey and his neighbors. Halsey, who bought land in the area after admiring it from the ferry on his commute between Flushing and Manhattan, had the village of Astoria incorporated in 1839. He named it after John Jacob Astor, just like the town in Oregon that Halsey's brother John had founded on a fur-trading expedition financed by Astor (the multimillionaire never went to either Astoria).

● Use the southeast exit from the station and walk straight ahead on 31st St. Through-out Astoria, you will find survivors from the 19th or early 20th century sandwiched between newer buildings of a vastly different character. On your left, for instance, see the house just past the five-story apartment building with balconies. It dates to the early 1910s; the brick town house next to it is a few years older. Farther down the block, a cute old-fashioned country church now has the elevated train pressed up against it and Chinese characters pressed onto it. It was built in the 1860s for a German congregation.

● Turn right on 30th Dr., bringing you to the front doors of St. Demetrios, the first Greek Orthodox church organized in Queens. In the 1980s, this church was elevated to cathedral and its pastor promoted to bishop.

● Turn right on 30th St. The Academy for New Americans, on your left, is a public mid-dle school that immigrant children attend for only one year. In addition to teaching them English (and other subjects), the school helps acculturate students and provides counseling services to aid in their transition.

- Turn left on 30th Ave. Athens Square, on your right, holds two gifts from Greece: a statue of Athena, presented by the mayor of Athens on behalf of his city, and a bust of Aristotle that came from the people of Chalcidice, a Macedonian region. They were placed in this space, designed to resemble a Greek amphitheater, alongside a bronze Socrates and a series of columns copied from a Delphi temple. The NYC leg of the Olympic torch relay preceding the 2004 Summer Games in Athens began, fittingly, at this park.

  At the corner of 29th St., Il Fornaio began as an Italian bakery (with an espresso bar) but has diversified, with cupcakes, rugelach, and a best-selling strudel among its plentiful goodies. From the bakery, walk one block on 29th St.

- Make a right on 30th Rd. At Crescent St., you're facing a throwback to rural Astoria, the 1868 Church of the Redeemer. To continue on 30th Rd., go left on Crescent St. and then make a quick right, walking alongside another church, now known as Good Shepherd United Methodist. The former First Methodist Episcopal has become an important cultural venue since 2008, when the Astoria Performing Arts Center (APAC) set up its main stage inside. APAC has continually garnered greater attention from theatergoers and critics, attracting Broadway veterans to perform in its shows and winning numerous off-Broadway awards for its productions.

- Turn right on 23rd St.

- Make a right on 30th Ave. The HANAC building, on your right, is still recognizable as a circa-1890 police station, thanks to its intact Romanesque detail and the police badges sculpted in the spandrel panels beneath top-floor windows. (HANAC, a social-services organization, was founded as the Hellenic American Neighborhood Action Committee.)

- Turn left on Crescent St. The Astoria Center of Israel, on your right after you pass 29th Ave., is one of Queens' oldest synagogues with an active congregation—though it had dwindled to about 100 members by the time the shul earned a spot on the National Register of Historic Places in 2009, the same year it held its first wedding in more than two decades. Inside are murals by French Art Deco artist Louis Rigal (whose work adorns the lobby of the Waldorf-Astoria) inspired by a passage in the Talmud, while the building's exterior artistry includes carved door panels depicting objects such as a menorah and kiddush cup. Another point of pride: The Astoria Center of Israel's rabbi when this building was constructed in the mid-1920s became the first Jewish chaplain of the US Navy during World War II.

● Go two more blocks to reach Our Lady of Mount Carmel Church, a massive limestone beauty. It was the first Catholic parish in Queens, begun around 1840. This is the church's second home, completed in 1873 but redesigned and enlarged in 1916.

● Turn left on Newtown Ave. On your left is the church's lovely parish hall, the Mount Carmel Institute. On your right, a public girls' school emphasizing math, science, and technology in its curriculum opened inside Mount Carmel's former school (which closed after 115 years in 2005).

Proceed on Newtown to where it joins Astoria Blvd. at 21st St. The Queens version of the Flatiron Building, surmounted by an onion-dome cupola, stands on a triangular lot across the street. Once entirely commercial, the building is now residential on upper floors.

● Cross 21st St. and go left onto Astoria Blvd., walking between the "flatiron" and the Astoria Islamic Center, founded by Bangladeshis. Astoria's Muslim population has increased by at least 80% since 1990. (Other mosques in the neighborhood have predominantly North African

Our Lady of Mount Carmel

DON'T FORGET THE STEINWAYS!

In addition to Stephen Halsey's village, Astoria holds remnants of another 19th-century village, the one developed by the Steinway family after they opened a factory, where the nonpareil pianos are handcrafted to this day. Brick row houses built in 1874–75 for Steinway & Sons employees can be found on 41st St. between 20th and 21st Aves. and on 20th Ave. in both directions off 41st St., with the original street names (Winthrop Ave., Albert St., and Theodore St.—the Steinway sons' names) inscribed on the corner buildings. A Reformed church built in 1890 on William Steinway's dime still stands at 41st St. and Ditmars Blvd. The Steinways also established a range of public services, including a streetcar line, library, public bathhouse, kindergarten, post office, and volunteer fire department, and even developed an amusement park and beer garden on Bowery Bay (where LaGuardia Airport is now) for workers to enjoy in their time off. The family's 27-room river-view villa incongruously survives at the northern end of 41st St., surrounded by body shops, manufacturers, and a power plant.

At the time Steinway was building its company town, piano making was a top-10 industry in New York. Of the 170 piano manufacturers NYC had at its peak in the 1870s, only Steinway remains. The factory, on 38th St. off 19th Ave., opens for a free public tour on Tuesday mornings (reservations required) that takes you through every step of a Steinway piano's creation, from the cutting of veneers to final tuning. You'll visit the mill where piano components are manufactured, the hot room where rims are aged, and the departments where new pianos receive their finishing and old pianos are restored.

memberships, and Steinway St. between Astoria Blvd. and 28th Ave. has been dubbed Little Egypt.) At the right corner with 14th St. is the first Queens library to be built with a grant from Andrew Carnegie, who funded the construction of thousands of libraries nationwide that were incorporated into public library systems. It dates from 1904.

Diagonally across 14th St., a chimneylike brick structure displays a memorial to three firemen, all fathers, killed in the line of duty on Father's Day 2001, a tragedy overshadowed three months later by the FDNY's massive loss on 9/11. The firefighters are also honored in a mural across the street. For a pick-me-up after this poignant sight, stop in the Astor Bake Shop, across 14th St. from the library.

- Walk north on 14th St., with the library to your right. You are now within the confines of the original Astoria village, which still has a decent concentration of 19th-century houses. Without landmark protection, however, every year it loses some of the old homes—usually replaced by bland or boxy multiunit dwellings. One example is visible just a few steps uphill: The historic cemetery belongs to St. George's, but the church and its graveyard now have a large modern building between them. That the new building contains low-income apartments for seniors did little to assuage disappointment over the destruction of the 1840 parsonage, which the financially strapped church sold to stay afloat. Turn your attention to what has survived; St. George's Church certainly does its best to transport you back to Astoria's days as a rural village. Established in 1827, it's one of the neighborhood's oldest institutions. This building went up in 1903 after a fire destroyed the original wooden house of worship, which was where the library is. Be sure to look up at the gargoyles.

- Cross 27th Ave. to continue on 14th St. To your right on the next block, a beautifully maintained duotone Queen Anne with delightful exterior decor serves as a salve against the new buildings beside it (another stylized vintage home was destroyed to make room for them). The black-and-white house's neighbor on the other side has some cute touches too, like its sunburst and oval window. Over on the left is an array of polygonal roofs and towers. The property on the right corner recalls Astoria village in its heyday, when lumber and shipping tycoons built large homes on spacious, elevated plots.

- Turn right on 26th Ave., where some old row houses survive on your left.

- Make a left on 14th Pl. This narrow road may very well have been designed in the 1800s for the carriage houses (i.e., garages) of 14th St. mansions. Today, it offers a great view of one tower of the Robert F. Kennedy Bridge, which links Astoria with Manhattan and the Bronx—hence the bridge's original name, Triborough, which everybody still calls it.

- At Astoria Park S., cross over the street and enter Astoria Park. Go to the right on the path, walking beside the running track, past the tennis courts, and then under the bridge. Proceed straight onto the path just inside the park, parallel to 19th St.

- Opposite 23rd Terr., descend the stairs on your left and onto the roof of the glass-block-walled bathhouse—though you can first go down the other steps to see the Art Deco bathhouse itself. This entire pool complex, from the cast-iron fence to the changing rooms to the flying-saucer-esque filter house, has been landmarked. It is the largest pool in a city park and was the largest Works Progress Administration (WPA) project in New York City other than Rockaway's Jacob Riis Park. Most park pools don't have such extensive bleacher seating; then again, they didn't need it like this pool did, since it hosted the US Olympic team trials for swimming and diving in 1936 and 1964. The diving pool has been out of commission for a while, but there are plans to transform it into an amphitheater-like performance space.

  The Triborough Bridge opened nine days after the pool in July 1936; meanwhile, the Hell Gate Bridge to your right, which carries only trains, has been around since 1917. It was the longest steel arch bridge in the world when built and inspired the design of Australia's Sydney Harbour Bridge. Hell Gate is the body of water it spans—a notoriously treacherous strait that caused so many shipwrecks that the US Army Corps of Engineers blasted out underwater rocks in the 1870s and 1880s, in explosions surpassed in magnitude only by the atomic bomb.

- Leave the pool viewing deck on the Triborough Bridge side, going down the stairs and onto the path. Follow it all the way downhill, between the pool and basketball courts, to Shore Blvd. On your right, a World War I memorial depicts an angel holding a sword in one hand and a laurel wreath (a symbol of peace and victory) in the other. Across the street, read about the *General Slocum*—other than 9/11, NYC's worst disaster ever in terms of loss of life—on the sign at the water's edge.

- Go south on Shore Blvd., passing beneath the Triborough Bridge again, and make a left when you're back at Astoria Park S.

- Turn right on 14th St. This block has been depleted of its historic homes, except for #25-37 on your left, which dates to 1852. Its parking lot used to be a large, lush lawn, and the house had a full-width balcony on the second floor with both Corinthian and Doric columns.

- Turn right on 26th Ave., then left on 12th St. The first house on your right is a fine Civil War–era model. But it's the property across the street that's recaptured the splendor of old Astoria like none other. This circa-1840 mansion is called Tara, à la Scarlett O'Hara's home in *Gone with the Wind,* and its grounds have been decked out like a Florentine villa. Continuing uphill, you'll find pre-1890s houses on both sides of the block that have eluded bad remodeling if not bright-colored paint. A Greek Orthodox church has converted an 1860s mansion on the left corner, across from a mid-1840s house (which fronts 27th Ave.) that's noted for the pairs of tiny windows lined up under the roof. On the next block, beneath a multispire verdigris steeple, the First Reformed Church is full of pointed arches, stained glass, brick, and terra-cotta. This 1888 Victorian Gothic classic is the second building for the congregation, which has had serious money woes just like the neighborhood's other historic church, St. George's.

● Turn right on Astoria Blvd. When it splits, go to the left, which is Main Ave. Fork left at the entrance to the community garden to stay on Main.

● Turn left across 8th St., which becomes Vernon Blvd. Past the playground, go right onto the waterfront path for some great vistas, then return to Vernon Blvd. and continue south. You're walking alongside Hallet's Cove, named for William Hallet, an Englishman who first made his home here in the 1650s. You can see the lighthouse on Roosevelt Island, an 1872 project by James Renwick Jr., architect of St. Patrick's Cathedral and the Smithsonian Institution.

Across from the water at 31st Ave., residences have been developed inside the landmarked former Sohmer piano factory, an unusually handsome industrial building, thanks to its clock tower and ornamented cupola. Sohmer had followed piano maker Steinway & Sons to Astoria but focused more on uprights for the home rather than grand pianos for the concert hall (though Sohmer was the first US firm to market baby grands). The company had its famous fans, including Irving Berlin, who composed on a Sohmer.

● Just south, go into Socrates Sculpture Park, a masterstroke of waterfront reclamation. The sculpture on exhibit ranges from representational to highly conceptual. Artists spearheaded the transformation of a dumping ground into this outdoor museum, whose on-site programming includes yoga sessions, film screenings, and kayaking on summer Sundays—all free to the public. The historic name for this area is Ravenswood, never a village as much as a 19th-century enclave of waterfront mansions. When Long Island City incorporated in 1870, it absorbed Ravenswood and Astoria village.

- Back on Vernon, make a left onto 10th St., then a right on 33rd Rd. for the entrance to the Noguchi Museum, which presents the work of acclaimed Japanese American sculptor Isamu Noguchi in a converted industrial building redesigned by the artist, who had a studio across the street from 1960 until his death in 1988. While Noguchi is best known for sculpture and public projects, such as Hiroshima's Peace Park and the UNESCO gardens in Paris, the full range of his work—extending to drawings, furniture and set design, and illuminated objects—are shown in the museum's indoor galleries and open-air sculpture garden.

- Upon leaving the museum, go back to Vernon Blvd. and Broadway, across from Socrates Sculpture Park, and take the Sunnyside-bound Q104 on Broadway to the N train at 31st St. (or walk the 0.6 mile).

POINTS OF INTEREST

Athens Square 30th Ave. and 29th St.
Il Fornaio Bakery 29-14 30th Ave., 718-267-0052
Astoria Performing Arts Center apacny.org, 30-44 Crescent St., 718-706-5750
Astor Bake Shop astor-bakeshop.com, 12-23 Astoria Blvd., 718-606-8439
Astoria Park 19th St. and 23rd Terr.
Socrates Sculpture Park socratessculpturepark.org, 32-01 Vernon Blvd., 718-956-1819
Noguchi Museum noguchi.org, 9-01 33rd Rd., 718-204-7088

route summary

1. Walk south on 31st St. from 30th Ave.
2. Turn right on 30th Dr.
3. Turn right on 30th St.
4. Make a left on 30th Ave.
5. Turn left on 29th St.
6. Make a right on 30th Rd., then left on Crescent St. and right to continue on 30th Rd.
7. Turn right on 23rd St.
8. Make a right on 30th Ave.
9. Turn left on Crescent St.
10. Turn left on Newtown Ave.
11. Bear left onto Astoria Blvd. across 21st St.
12. Turn right on 14th St.
13. Make a right on 26th Ave.
14. Make a left on 14th Pl.
15. Cross Astoria Park S. and go into the park, eventually exiting onto Shore Blvd.
16. Turn left on Astoria Park S., then right on 14th St.
17. Turn right on 26th Ave.
18. Make a left on 12th St.
19. Turn right on Astoria Blvd., which branches off to Main Ave.
20. At 8th St., go left onto Vernon Blvd.
21. Go down and back along the waterfront path.
22. Make a left from Vernon Blvd. on 10th St. and right on 33rd Rd.
23. Walk back to Broadway for the bus or walk to the N train station at 31st St.

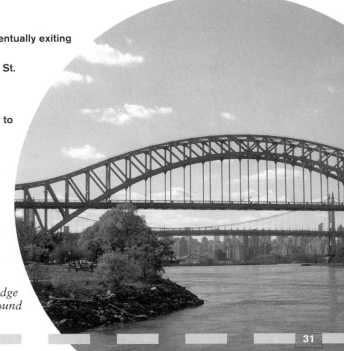

The Hell Gate Bridge, with the Triborough Bridge in the background

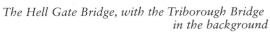

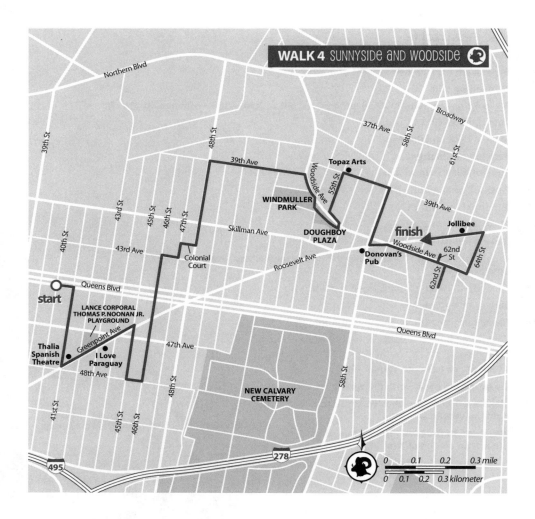

Northern Blvd

Broadway

37th Ave

58th St

61st St

48th St

39th Ave

Topaz Arts

Woodside Ave

55th St

39th Ave

43rd St

45th St

46th St

47th St

WINDMULLER
PARK

Skillman Ave

Jollibee

DOUGHBOY
PLAZA

finish

39th St

40th St

43rd Ave

Colonial
Court

Roosevelt Ave

Donovan's
Pub

Woodside Ave

62nd
St

64th St

62nd St

start

Queens Blvd

LANCE CORPORAL
THOMAS P. NOONAN JR.
PLAYGROUND

Queens Blvd

Greenpoint Ave

47th Ave

58th St

Thalia
Spanish
Theatre

I Love
Paraguay

48th Ave

48th St

NEW CALVARY
CEMETERY

41st St

45th St

46th St

495

278

0   0.1   0.2   0.3 mile

0   0.1   0.2   0.3 kilometer

4 SUNNYSIDE AND WOODSIDE: THINK GLOBAL, LIVE LOCAL

BOUNDARIES: **39th Ave., 64th St., 48th Ave., 40th St.**
DISTANCE: **3 miles**
SUBWAY: **7 to 40th St.**

Situated side by side along the 7 line, Sunnyside and Woodside are quintessentially Queens. Within these melting pots, you'll find NYC's Little Manila, the Islamic Institute of New York, an Ecuador Consulate office (the only one any country has opened outside Manhattan), a cluster of Romanian shops and restaurants, and what many consider the city's best Thai restaurant, SriPraPhai—to name but a few examples of their immense diversity. Yet they're considered Irish neighborhoods, as you'll deduce from all the pubs this route passes. Woodside was 80% Irish at one time, while Sunnyside used to be home base for the Irish-American Athletic Club, whose former property is now the Celtic Park apartments. You might think the two neighborhoods arose together, but they didn't. Woodside was a place of country manors before real estate speculators and railroad service arrived in the 1860s, and it eventually absorbed a town called Winfield that had developed earlier. Sunnyside, once part of Long Island City, only began to flourish in the 1910s and '20s with the opening of the bridge, the subway, and the planned community of Sunnyside Gardens.

● In the 40th St. station, platforms and turnstile areas are adorned with letters *K* through *P* of the *Q Is for Queens* art installation, stained glass windows depicting aspects of Queens history or culture by letter. That's the Onderdonk House in Ridgewood on the *O* window, for instance; Corona's Langston Hughes Library celebrated in *L;* and the moviemaking that's taken place at Astoria studios in *M.* (The rest of the alphabet can be found at the 33rd and 46th St. stations.)

● Exit on the southeast corner of Queens Blvd. and 40th St., and cross over to the sidewalk. From there, you can appreciate another artistic feature of the 7 train: polychromatic terra-cotta decorating the concrete viaduct. Walk east on Queens Blvd. (that is, with Manhattan behind you).

- Turn right on 41st St., also known as Benjamin Wheeler Pl. Benjamin, one of the children killed at Sandy Hook Elementary School, lived on this street as a baby, before his family moved to Newtown, Connecticut. At 47th Ave., you have a great view of the Empire State Building, and at the next intersection, Greenpoint Ave., the tall steeple to your right belongs to St. Raphael Roman Catholic Church (1885), which originated as the mortuary chapel for Calvary Cemetery, the country's largest cemetery in number of burials (about 3 million).

- Make a left on Greenpoint Ave. On your left, Thalia Spanish Theatre has been presenting bilingual plays since 1977. At the next corner, enter Lance Corporal Thomas P. Noonan Jr. Playground at the eagle imprint, and walk on the botanical-themed pavement parallel to the avenue. This park, named for an Irish American Medal of Honor winner, is where the Turkish Cultural Center sets up its Ramadan tent. Note the halal Chinese restaurant across Greenpoint Ave. Leave the park via the steps at 43rd St., where an eagle medallion is posted on the fence. The eagles come from the insignia of the US Marines, in which Noonan served during the Vietnam War.

  On the next block of Greenpoint Ave., just past the library, you can grab an empanada or an entire meal at I Love Paraguay, or I Love Py, as it's often called. Stay to the left at 44th St. to remain on Greenpoint Ave. The building on your left at 45th St. has been a Jehovah's Witnesses Assembly Hall longer than it was a cinema—the 2,000-seat Bliss theater, which opened around 1931 with Egyptian-inspired ornamentation. Jehovah's Witnesses, who took over the property in the 1960s, have maintained the exterior but eradicated most of the theater's interior decor because the Egypt-history murals showed nudity and pagan symbols.

- Make a right on 45th St., passing between two apartment buildings with contrasting types of Tudor facades—half-timbering on your right, brick-accented stucco on your left—on the far side of 47th Ave.

- Turn left on 48th Ave., which encapsulates the amazing diversity of Queens on a single block containing an Irish pub, a Mexican restaurant, churches with Korean- and Spanish-speaking congregations, a mosque, and a Romanian Orthodox church. The beautiful mosaics around the latter's doorway deserve a closer look.

● Go left on 46th St. Three blocks away, you walk beneath the kitschy yet welcoming Sunnyside arch as you head across Queens Blvd. North of the boulevard, a plaque beside the door of 43-30 46th St. remembers Bix Beiderbecke, the jazz musician who'd been living in Apartment 1G for a little more than a month when he died there at the age of 28, of pneumonia aggravated by heavy drinking. Beiderbecke's death did not make the news, but his legend grew posthumously, and today he is recognized as an important and influential figure in jazz. Every year, around the anniversary of his death, Sunnyside hosts a daylong memorial concert. Next door are the garden and church of All Saints Episcopal, formed in the 1920s to serve the original residents of Sunnyside Gardens. Korean, South Indian, and Latino congregations also hold services at the church now. Sunny Grocery, on your left at 43rd Ave., not only sells Turkish foods but also functions as an unofficial welcome center for Turkish immigrants.

● Turn right on 43rd Ave. Down the block on your right, you can see into the backyard of Wilson Court, one of the 11 Sunnyside Gardens properties. Created in the 1920s, Sunnyside Gardens was the first practical application of concepts espoused by the Regional Planning Association of America (RPAA), formed to generate ideas for higher-quality working-class housing. RPAA's members included Clarence Stein and Henry Wright, the architects of Sunnyside Gardens. Most of its developments (row houses as well as low-rise apartment buildings) were constructed around a full block, with a common garden, or court, behind the buildings. Wilson Court, though, does not extend around a whole block's perimeter; it comprises this corner building on the avenue and seven adjoining buildings going down 47th. Opposite them, on the east side of the street, is another Sunnyside Gardens complex, Carolin Gardens, which takes its name from 47th St.'s former moniker. Street signs within the Sunnyside Gardens historic district show both the original names and the numbers by which streets and avenues are currently known.

● Turn left on 47th St. This entire block, including the houses along 43rd Ave., is occupied by Colonial Court, the first project completed in Sunnyside Gardens. As designed, no house in any of the developments had an individual backyard, and their gardens were public.

- Turn right into the alley between #41-35 and #41-31. Originally, the green space to your right was open to all Colonial Court's residents, but it was divided into private backyards after land easements expired. A common greensward remains on your left.

- Turn left onto 48th St. The row houses on the east side of the block are not part of Sunnyside Gardens but also raised the standard of living for the working class. More than 1,000 of these Mathews Model Flats were built in Queens, primarily Ridgewood, between 1905 and 1930.

  Meanwhile, on the Colonial Court side of the street, an original resident of #41-12 was Lewis Mumford, the architecture critic and urban historian. Mumford was involved in the RPAA with Sunnyside Gardens' creators and was quoted extensively in promotional material for the community. He lived here briefly before moving to Madison Court on 44th St., where he resided for a decade. Sunnyside Gardens was inspired by England's garden city movement, but unlike older Queens communities planned on that model, it was not conceived or marketed as upscale. It served as a model for developments nationwide and is credited with laying the groundwork for the New Urbanism movement that took hold decades later.

  Across Skillman Ave., the Sunnyside Reformed Church fits right into Sunnyside Gardens, though it predates the neighborhood. On this block, you have nicely landscaped Jefferson Court on your right, and you can go up the steps for a better look at its unconventional layout: U-shaped arrangements of row houses, which are entered off-street and have communal gardens in front rather than back. On your left, the houses of Roosevelt Court have slate tiles on the gabled roofs and parapets along the flat rooflines. If you'd like to see more of the gardens, take a pathway through Roosevelt Court to 47th St. so you can see behind the homes, then return to 48th and continue north.

- Turn right on 39th Ave. All the row houses on this avenue from 47th to 52nd St. belong to Harrison Place. Only the ones on your right and those along 48th and 49th Sts., which form a U with them, had a common back lawn, but it's been divvied up into private yards. On your left, opposite 49th, is Sunnyside Gardens Park, the only private park in New York City other than über-exclusive Gramercy Park on Manhattan's east side. This one is larger and, because it's not enclosed by locked gates like

Gramercy, less foreboding to outsiders, not to mention more affordable and convivial for members—who lower their dues by putting in volunteer hours.

● Continue on 39th Ave. Past 50th St. on your left is Phipps Garden Apartments, built separately from Sunnyside Gardens but part of the historic district. Even the fire escapes on this early 1930s complex have an Art Deco style. The same team that created Sunnyside Gardens designed the Phipps buildings and grounds, which include a landscaped interior courtyard.

● Turn right on Woodside Ave., crossing into Woodside. At 54th St., go up the stairs on your right into Windmuller Park, the former locale of Hillside Manor, the summer home of banker Louis Windmuller and his family. The Windmuller property, whose grounds were landscaped by Central Park designer Frederick Law Olmsted, was one of the last surviving Woodside estates, as part of it wasn't sold off to developers until the 1940s.

● Make a left on the street (39th Dr.) after walking through the sitting area, turn a corner, and go down the steps on your left. A ramp takes you into Doughboy Plaza. The wall and garden to your right memorialize Woodside's 9/11 losses, among them firefighter Lawrence Virgilio, for whom the playground is now named in this park where he played as a child. The *Returning Soldier,* as the plaza's eponymous statue is formally named, pays tribute to the local men who died fighting World War I. It won a national prize for war memorials in the 1920s. The soldier is not in the midst of combat but finished with service, his

The Woodside Doughboy

head bandaged and his expression conveying the toll of battle—a far less bombastic expression of valor than many war monuments.

- Behind the Doughboy, exit the park down the steps and onto 55th St. Walk one block and turn right on 39th Ave. The first nonresidential building on your left, #55-03, is Topaz Arts, which has created both a gallery and a dance studio inside a former warehouse; pay a visit if it's open. Then continue east on 39th Ave. Some of the buildings reveal Woodside history under layers of modifications. On your left at 57th St., for example, the corner home has three top-floor windows with shutters on both the avenue and street sides—just as it did when it was a roadhouse named the Woodside Pavilion in 1880. A onetime employee, John Meyer, opened his own hotel a block away: The house on your left across 58th St., virtually underneath the train tracks, was Meyer's Hotel, advertised as "first class" and "opposite the depot." Woodside's rail station was located at 58th St. and 38th Ave. until 1915, when it was moved to 61st St. and Roosevelt Ave. for a direct connection with the new subway.

- Turn right and head south on 58th St. On your right at the next intersection, St. Sebastian School occupies the approximate site of the Kelly estate that gave Woodside its name. Journalist John A. Kelly published a series of "Letters from Woodside" in the Brooklyn newspaper he co-owned (the name Sunnyside, meanwhile, is believed to have originated with a tavern popular with horse-racing fans). St. Sebastian built its first church at this location in 1896.

- Cross Woodside Ave. and then Roosevelt Ave. to reach the current St. Sebastian's Church. Is there something about it, particularly its windowless 58th St. side, that doesn't quite look like a church? That's because it was built as a movie palace, the Loew's Woodside, which had a Wurlitzer organ and orchestra to accompany the films when it opened in 1926. The 2,000-seat cinema was designed by Herbert J. Krapp, architect of more than a dozen extant Broadway theaters. Across the street from the church, neighborhood mainstay Donovan's Pub has topped a number of best-burger-in-New York lists.

- Walk east on Roosevelt Ave., with the church to your right.

- Stay to the right so that you're on Woodside Ave. as you pass the second triangular park. The 1927 bank building on your right at 60th St. has imposing Corinthian columns.

- Turn left on 62nd St. Abutting the Long Island Rail Road platform on the left is an attractive apartment building, Woodside Court, that happens to be the neighborhood's earliest, erected in 1916. As there's nowhere else to go from here, turn around, go back to Woodside Ave., and make a left.

  Turn right to continue on 62nd St. Buildings on the right past the apartments were the campus of a watchmaking school that Bulova established for disabled World War II veterans. Mayor Fiorello LaGuardia laid the cornerstone, still visible at the lower right of the cupolaed building (now a Mormon center). Bulova's school existed into the 1990s, long enough to enroll vets of Korea and Vietnam and open up to disabled civilians too. Physical therapy and other services were provided on-site.

- Return to Woodside Ave. and make a right in front of the Queens Landmark condominium, which occupies the former Bulova factory (the company is still headquartered in Queens).

  Turn left on 64th St. On your right, #39-73 is believed to have been an inn in the mid-19th century. It matches photos and the location of a Shaw's Hotel of the 1840s, which would make it one of Woodside's oldest buildings. Local history buffs fear it will be razed for development.

- Make a left at Roosevelt Ave. Jollibee, on the right at 63rd St., is a Filipino fast-food chain—signature dish: fried chicken—that had hundreds of restaurants in the Philippines and more than 20 on the West Coast before opening this New York City location. This is the west end of Little Manila, some 10 blocks around Roosevelt Ave. where Filipino businesses and organizations are concentrated and the Bayanihan Cultural Festival is held every year.

- Continue west on Roosevelt Ave. to 61st St. for the 7 train.

POINTS OF INTEREST

Thalia Spanish Theatre thaliatheatre.org, 41-17 Greenpoint Ave., 718-729-3880

Lance Corporal Thomas P. Noonan Jr. Playground Greenpoint Ave. and 42nd St.

I Love Paraguay ilovepy.com, 43-16 Greenpoint Ave., 718-786-5534

Windmuller Park Woodside Ave. and 54th St.

Doughboy Plaza Woodside Ave. and 56th St.

Topaz Arts topazarts.org, 55-03 39th Ave., 718-505-0440

Donovan's Pub donovansny.com, 57-24 Roosevelt Ave., 718-429-9339

Jollibee jollibeeusa.com, 62-29 Roosevelt Ave., 718-426-4445

route summary

1. From Queens Blvd. and 40th St., walk east.
2. Turn right on 41st St.
3. Turn left on Greenpoint Ave.
4. Make a right on 45th St.
5. Go left on 48th Ave.
6. Turn left on 46th St.
7. Turn right on 43rd Ave.
8. Make a left on 47th St.
9. Take the Colonial Court alley to 48th St., and go left.
10. Turn right on 39th Ave.
11. Make a right on Woodside Ave.
12. Walk in Windmuller Park and adjacent Doughboy Plaza.
13. Head north on 55th St.
14. Turn right on 39th Ave.
15. Make a right on 58th St.
16. Turn left on Roosevelt Ave., then fork right onto Woodside Ave.
17. Go in and out of 62nd St. on your left, and then proceed on Woodside Ave.
18. Go partway down 62nd St. to your right, and then return to Woodside Ave. and continue east.
19. Make a left on 64th St.
20. Go left on Roosevelt Ave. to 61st St.

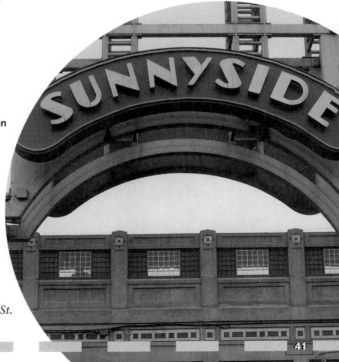

The arch and 7 train station at 46th St.

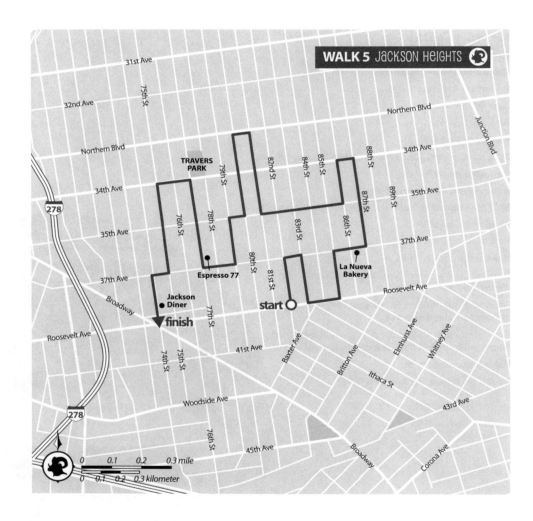

WALK 5 JACKSON HEIGHTS

31st Ave

32nd Ave

75th St

Northern Blvd

Northern Blvd

TRAVERS PARK

79th St

34th Ave

82nd St

84th St

85th St

88th St

34th Ave

89th St

35th Ave

278

34th Ave

76th St

78th St

35th Ave

83rd St

87th St

86th St

37th Ave

Espresso 77

80th St

La Nueva Bakery

37th Ave

81st St

Roosevelt Ave

Jackson Diner

start

Broadway

77th St

finish

Baxter Ave

Britton Ave

Elmhurst Ave

Whitney Ave

Roosevelt Ave

41st Ave

Ithaca St

74th St

75th St

43rd Ave

Woodside Ave

76th St

45th Ave

Broadway

Corona Ave

278

0   0.1   0.2   0.3 mile

0   0.1   0.2   0.3 kilometer

5 JaCKSON HeiGHTS: DiVErSITY BLOOMS IN a GarDeN COMMUNITY

BOUNDARIES: Northern Blvd., 87th St., Roosevelt Ave., 74th St.
DISTANCE: 3 miles
SUBWAY: 7 to 82nd St.

Current residents of Jackson Heights benefit from thoughtful urban planning of a century ago. The Queensboro Corporation created Jackson Heights around 1910, taking inspiration from England's garden city movement. Queensboro president Edward A. MacDougall envisioned an alternative to the typical high-density housing of the day, those dark, cramped tenements with poor ventilation that filled concrete-dominated neighborhoods. In Jackson Heights, residences would be set back from sidewalks, and only half the land in an apartment complex would actually be built on. The results were so-called garden apartments, each complex encompassing a private park for residents. The city has designated Jackson Heights a historic district, which prohibits major exterior alterations or new construction that's out of character. Thus, the gracious-living ethos on which Jackson Heights was founded still pervades its residential streets. Yet one important thing is different nowadays. The Queensboro Corporation created a restricted community, with an approval process for prospective residents, which kept out nonwhites. Today, however, Jackson Heights is one of the most diverse places in the world, with a large Indian community centered on 74th St. and a Latino majority overall.

● **Exit on the north side of Roosevelt Ave. and walk straight ahead on 82nd St. What may look like a run-of-the-mill shopping strip at first glance features distinguished storefronts starting about halfway down the block on the left and wrapping around the avenue. They were built in 1928 as part of the Queensboro Corporation's design for Jackson Heights. The original shopkeepers were subject to Queensboro's approval of their signage and merchandise displays. The corporation had its headquarters in the corner building, now a bank, with ram's heads flanking the doors.**

● **Turn right on 37th Ave., then right on 83rd St. On the left, you have your first look at a typical garden-apartment complex by the Queensboro Corporation: Its buildings line two adjacent streets (in this case, 83rd and 84th) and share the greensward** between them. What's atypical about this one, the Spanish Gardens, is the Spanish Baroque decorative elements at the top. On your right, the 8 brick row houses are the only survivors of 24 built in 1911 on 83rd and 82nd Sts., the first residences constructed by the Queensboro Corporation in the neighborhood.

● Make a left on Roosevelt Ave.

● Turn left on 85th St. The Queensboro Corporation introduced cooperative home ownership (whereby apartment buyers get a stake in the building ownership) to the borough with Linden Court, on the left, in 1919. Linden Court also attracted attention for its design: The corporation's new architect Andrew J. Thomas opted for unattached buildings and included garages. You can peek into the garden through the gates between buildings. Across the street is Cambridge Court, the last Jackson Heights apartments by Queensboro's original architect, George H. Wells, who designed the corporation's first 6 developments and more than 10 total.

● Turn right on 37th Ave. La Nueva Bakery, an Uruguayan café at #86-10, has an incredible selection of bread, snacks, and desserts (*postres*), including some Argentinean and Colombian specialties. The elementary school farther down the block is named in honor of Christopher Santora, the youngest firefighter killed on 9/11. The son of an FDNY deputy chief, 23-year-old Santora lived in Queens his entire life and joined the fire department just two months before the attacks.

● Make a left on 87th St. In the mid-1920s, having developed more than 15 apartment buildings, the Queensboro Corporation added houses to the mix, and this was the first street to get them. The company spent liberally on high-quality craftsmanship and materials. The dwellings were dubbed English Garden Homes and built in attached pairs, like on the left, and longer rows, like on your right.

● Crossing 35th Ave., you pass a low Salvation Army building on your left—it's all that was constructed of a grand structure planned for the First Church of Christ, Scientist that was to be several stories tall and fronted by a triangular pediment and Ionic columns. But the congregation ran out of money after this ground floor was finished in 1927. The larger structure with a rounded glass front next to it was the eventual completion—25 years later—of the church. There are more English Garden Homes to admire past 35th Ave.

- Turn left on 34th Ave.

- Turn left on 86th St. Before the neighborhood was landmarked, developers bought out several homeowners, which explains how blah modern apartment buildings ended up on streets with the English Garden Homes. The last house on the left shows both its current and former (158 29th St.) addresses. Like many neighborhoods, Jackson Heights originally had its own street numbers and names, but streets were later renumbered to conform to Queens' overall grid.

- Turn right on 35th Ave. The left side of the next block has the Belvedere, a delight from the tips of its multiple towers down to its arcaded entry. It was designed by Joshua Tabatchnik, a favorite Queensboro Corporation architect of the 1930s. Across 84th St., mysterious figures guard the loggias atop Cedar Court on your right.

  Don't miss the street sign at 81st St. in front of Community United Methodist Church, the oldest house of worship in Jackson Heights. Those subscript numbers on 35TH AVENUE are the letters' Scrabble values, a tribute to the board game's birthplace. In the early 1930s, local resident Alfred M. Butts, an architect who'd been laid off because of the Great Depression, invented a game he called Lexiko and brought it to the church hall for people to play as he tested it out. Butts ultimately earned more than $1 million from his invention, but it took nearly two decades and heavy promotion by Macy's for the game to catch on. Butts resumed working as an architect, even designing the church's education building to the left.

- Turn right on 81st St. Most of the left side belongs to the Chateau, which entails 12 buildings and was modeled on the French Renaissance castles that inspired its name. When it opened in 1923, nobody thought it would ever be surpassed in opulence, and it still impresses with its slate mansard roofs, iron finials, and patterned brickwork on corner buildings.

- Cross 34th Ave. St. Mark's Episcopal Church, to your right, was designed by Robert Tappan, the architect responsible for most of the English Garden Homes. Standing opposite the Chateau is the Towers, which opened a year later and raised Jackson Heights' luxury bar even higher. Both were designed by Andrew J. Thomas.

With its posh interiors, the Towers was advertised as comparable to Park Ave., and Queensboro president Edward MacDougall himself moved in. Its eight buildings are spaced nearly 40 feet apart and occupy less than two-fifths of the land. Continue along 81st St. and look into the garden of the Towers, which holds a baldachino (a gazebo-type structure composed of columns and an ironwork canopy) in the middle and fountains at both ends.

- Make two lefts, looping around Northern Blvd. onto 80th St. Across from the Chateau is Elm Court, the first Jackson Heights apartments to have push-button elevators and one of three apartment complexes designed by George H. Wells that opened in 1922.

- Turn right on 35th Ave.

- Turn left on 79th St. On your right is 1921's Hampton Court, which Wells modeled after Harvard dormitories. It has different doorways and projecting bays on 78th St., a divergence from the neighborhood norm of uniform exteriors within a complex. The white building on your right at the end of the block—the last Jackson Heights design by Andrew J. Thomas—became the Queensboro Corporation's new headquarters in 1947, three years after the death of longtime president MacDougall.

- Turn right on 37th Ave. The school between 78th and 77th Sts. is flanked by honorary street names: Julio Rivera Corner at 78th and Edgar Garzon Corner on 77th. Both these men were killed in gay-bashing incidents (11 years apart) on the streets now named for them. Rivera's murder spurred the formation of the Queens Pride agency in Jackson Heights, which has traditionally been the gay center of Queens. The annual pride parade here is the largest in the city outside Greenwich Village.

- Turn right on 77th St. Espresso 77 on the right is known citywide among java aficionados and makes its own special flavors of lattes. The apartments on the left are Hawthorne Court, another of Wells's 1922 developments. More than a decade later, architect Joshua Tabatchnik maintained the Georgian ambience on the block with the Berkeley (on the right) and showed a fondness for urns.

- Proceed to 34th Ave. In the 1940s, when developers were buying up all open land, Jackson Heights residents lobbied the city to set aside space for a public park. Some 50 years later, residents brought Travers Park back from near ruin after it became a graffiti-scarred drug-dealer hangout. Concerned residents did much of the cleanup and gardening and formed a group, Friends of Travers Park, that brings entertainment and other special events to the park and advocates for green space in the neighborhood. Across 77th from the park are the castlelike Fairway apartments, constructed in the mid-1930s where a golf-course fairway had been. The design for Jackson Heights included a golf course, tennis courts, and clubhouse—though all these recreational facilities were gone by the time Travers Park came into being.

● Walk on 34th Ave. past the Fairway, and turn left on 75th St. The Spanish Towers, halfway down on your right, is a small group of attached houses that nonetheless commands attention with their Mediterranean style, overhanging tile roofs, and wood shutters.

● Turn right on 37th Ave. into a commercial district abounding with Indian eateries, sari shops, jewelers, and music stores. Take your pick of the food places; have a full meal, snack on a samosa or *dosa,* or satisfy a sweet craving with *mithai.* Some restaurants in the vicinity specialize in Himalayan cuisine.

● Turn left on 74th St. Jackson Diner, long regarded as the city's best Indian restaurant, is on the left. To the right, 37th Rd. off 74th St. has been closed to cars and turned into a proto–town commons called Diversity Plaza. Note the street sign here honoring Kalpana Chawla, the first Indian American astronaut, who died aboard the *Columbia* space shuttle. At Roosevelt Ave., you can catch the 7, E, F, R, or M subway.

POINTS OF INTEREST

La Nueva Bakery lanuevabakery.com, 86-10 37th Ave., 718-507-2339

Espresso 77 espresso77.com, 35-57 77th St., 718-424-1077

Travers Park 34th Ave. and 77th St.

Jackson Diner jacksondiner.com, 37-47 74th St., 718-672-1232

route summary

1. Walk north on 82nd St.
2. Turn right on 37th Ave.
3. Turn right on 83rd St.
4. Turn left on Roosevelt Ave.
5. Turn left on 85th St.
6. Turn right on 37th Ave.
7. Turn left on 87th St.
8. Turn left on 34th Ave.
9. Turn left on 86th St.
10. Turn right on 35th Ave.
11. Turn right on 81st St.
12. Turn left on Northern Blvd.
13. Go left on 80th St.
14. Turn right on 35th Ave.
15. Turn left on 79th St.
16. Make a right on 37th Ave.
17. Make a right on 77th St.
18. Turn left on 34th Ave.
19. Turn left on 75th St.
20. Turn right on 37th Ave.
21. Go left on 74th St. to Roosevelt Ave.

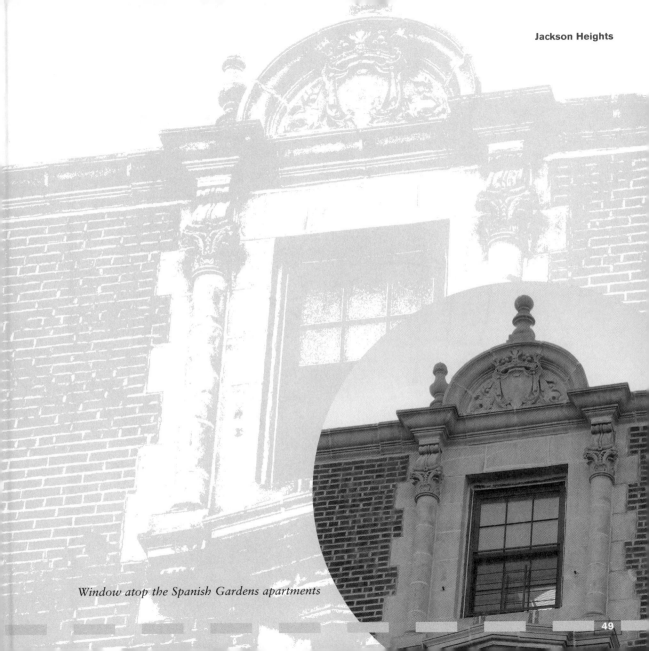

Window atop the Spanish Gardens apartments

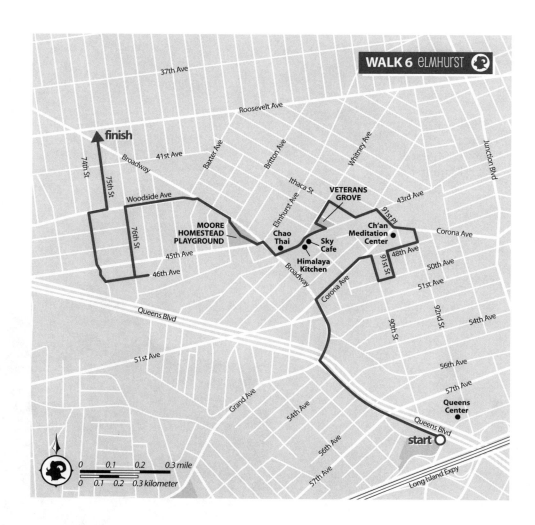

WALK 6 eLMHUrST

37th Ave

Roosevelt Ave

finish

74th St
75th St
Broadway
41st Ave
Baxter Ave
Britton Ave
Whitney Ave
Junction Blvd

Woodside Ave
Ithaca St
Elmhurst Ave
VETERANS GROVE
43rd Ave
91st Pl
Corona Ave

76th St
MOORE HOMESTEAD PLAYGROUND
Chao Thai
Sky Cafe
Ch'an Meditation Center

45th Ave
Himalaya Kitchen
Broadway
48th Ave
91st St
50th Ave

46th Ave
Corona Ave
51st Ave

Queens Blvd

90th St
92nd St
54th Ave

51st Ave
Grand Ave
56th Ave
57th Ave
Queens Center

54th Ave
Queens Blvd
start

56th Ave

57th Ave
Long Island Expy

0   0.1   0.2   0.3 mile
0   0.1   0.2   0.3 kilometer

6 ELMHURST: BACK TO THE FUTURE

BOUNDARIES: **Broadway, 92nd St., Queens Blvd., 74th St.**
DISTANCE: **3.2 miles**
SUBWAY: **R or M to Woodhaven Blvd.**

Reflecting on recent census figures, a local newspaper columnist wrote that Americans should look to Elmhurst for "what their future holds." The same thing could have been said in 1776. While many then living in Queens were loyal to their British homeland during the American Revolution, Elmhurst was a Patriot stronghold. And here we are, almost 250 years later, with the tenor in Elmhurst again expected to prevail nationwide. The newspaper columnist was referring to Elmhurst's status as a melting pot with a white minority, which is predicted for the overall US population within a few decades. The many houses of worship along this walk highlight not only Elmhurst's prodigious diversity but its long history too. Elmhurst grew out of one of the first European settlements in Queens, which was named Middleburg upon its founding in 1652 and rechristened Newtown in the 1680s. It kept that name until real estate developers began molding the rural village into a contemporary residential neighborhood in the late 1800s.

● Follow signs in the subway for Woodhaven Blvd. and Queens Blvd., and exit at their southwest corner, across from Queens Center, the middle of three suburban-style malls located along a 0.75-mile stretch of Queens Blvd. The names of Queens neighborhoods are banded around its midsection. Walk with the mall to your right. One long block away on your left, the Rock Church occupies a 1928 theater that ran the gamut from vaudeville house to multiplex over 70 years.

● Proceed to First Presbyterian at 54th Ave. The church was established circa 1652 by minister John Moore, a founder of Middleburg, and erected this building, its third, in 1893. In the 1920s, the building was moved back 125 feet when Queens Blvd. was widened; the steeple taken down for the project was never reinstalled. But those modifications were benign compared with the ransacking of First Presbyterian's original church by the British during the American Revolution.

● Go one more block to Grand Ave., and cross Queens Blvd.—with care. An unforgettable banner headline in the *Daily News* proclaimed Queens Blvd. the "Boulevard of

Death" in 2001 (73 pedestrians had been killed on it the preceding eight years), and while longer crossing times and other safety measures have been implemented, the 13 lanes can still pose a challenge.

- Walk on Broadway to 51st Ave. On your left is Old St. James Church, built in 1734, though it's undergone numerous alterations and hasn't been used for worship by the Episcopal congregation in years. At the next intersection is Old St. James's companion on the Elmhurst page in the National Register of Historic Places: the Reformed Church of Newtown, established by Dutch residents of the English settlement in the 1730s. This 1831 classic has a cornerstone from the church's original building.

- Turn right on Corona Ave., with St. James's present church on your left. On your right, the graves of some of the first families of Queens—Remsen, Suydam, Lent, Rapelye— are now squeezed between the Reformed Church's driveway and an auto body shop.

- After passing the Korean Evangelical Church, go right at the triangle onto 48th Ave. and then right on 90th St. beneath the multipeaked tower of Newtown High School. It's one of the masterpieces by C. B. J. Snyder, the city's longtime superintendent of school construction whose buildings were called "palaces of the people." Continue around the school via 50th Ave. and 91st St. to appreciate as much of this Flemish Renaissance Revival landmark as possible, with all the exquisite detail in its doorways, windows, and gables. There's been a school on this site since the 1860s, when children of all ages were taught in a plain wooden schoolhouse. Newtown High's alumni include actress Zoe Saldana, Kiss rocker Gene Simmons, *All in the Family* star Carroll O'Connor, cosmetics magnate Estée Lauder, opera star Risë Stevens, and comedian Don Rickles.

- Make a right from 91st St. back onto 48th Ave. Bethany Lutheran Church and its cutout tower exude some country charm at 91st Pl.

- Go left on 92nd St. one short block to Corona Ave., where the Hindu temple is bound to catch your eye. The late swami who established this temple—in a converted supermarket—also opened a large temple in neighboring Woodside.

- Turn left onto Corona Ave.

- Turn right on 91st Pl., which bridges the Long Island Rail Road tracks. As you head uphill, look back over your shoulder at the Ch'an Meditation Center on Corona Ave.

This Zen Buddhist organization hosts weekly chanting and meditation sessions open to the general public. On 91st Pl., the Chinese Lutheran church at #43-33, with columns and eagles, is recognizable as a former bank.

- Turn left on 43rd Ave., then right on Ithaca St. A Catholic church shares the block with a temple complex of Jainism. On your left, St. Bartholomew's rectory stands between its old and current sanctuaries. You are welcome to go inside the Jain Center on your right (the door's in the rear): Its fourth-floor temple contains a 13-foot-high, 7.5-ton shrine carved of crystal stones and holding gemstone idols within niches, and there are elaborately adorned temples on two other floors as well.

- Turn left on Whitney Ave., bringing you in front of the current St. Bartholomew. At the other end of the block, in the midst of all this modern urban multiculturalism, Elmhurst Baptist Church looks like something out of a Jane Austen novel. You can see from the signs that Elmhurst Baptist offers its premises to other faiths, as it has been doing throughout its 110-year history. Both St. Bartholomew and the Chinese church on the next block held services at Elmhurst Baptist before they had their own houses of worship. Across from that Chinese church, walk through Veterans Grove to see the park's complement on its 43rd Ave. side: the eagle-topped Elmhurst Memorial Hall, built for an American Legion post.

- Turn right on 43rd Ave. The row houses next to the veterans' hall were constructed in 1905, when Cord Meyer was developing Elmhurst. The real estate company purchased Newtown farmland in the 1890s, rechristened the place Elmhurst, planned its roads, created a sewer system, and brought in trolley service and retailers.

- At the tip of the triangle, resume walking on Whitney Ave. You can dine at an Indonesian (Sky Cafe) or Tibetan and Indian (Himalaya Kitchen) restaurant ahead on your left, or at the highly rated Chao Thai on the right. Or if you'd like to venture elsewhere in culinary Asia, there are Vietnamese, Malaysian, and other choices around the corner on Broadway.

- Turn right on Broadway. After crossing Elmhurst/45th Ave., enter Moore Homestead Playground. Go up the steps and walk between the comfort station and playground. Samuel Moore, son of First Presbyterian minister John Moore, built his estate here in 1661, and the Moore family owned the property until the 1930s. Clement C. Moore, Samuel's great-great-grandson, is believed to have spent much time here in his youth; he was a theologian (the family business) but is best remembered as the author of "The Night Before Christmas." The Newtown pippin, a tasty green apple that was immensely popular in the 18th and 19th centuries but is now all but forgotten, was first cultivated on the Moores' land. Thomas Jefferson obtained saplings for Monticello, and they were also planted at George Washington's home, Mount Vernon.

● Proceed through the park and exit at the corner of 82nd St. and Broadway. Continue west on Broadway.

● Go left onto Woodside Ave., across from Elmhurst Hospital. Its personnel speak more than 100 languages and can recognize medical conditions that might baffle doctors elsewhere in the United States because they're common only in certain foreign countries. On Woodside Ave. past 78th St., you're in the heart of Little Thailand, though Korean and Indonesian businesses also line the avenue, and Satya Narayan Mandir at the corner of 76th St. serves Sindhis, an ethnic group of Pakistan. In the Sindhi tradition, this temple combines Hindu and Sikh observances, and it may be the only *gurmandir* (*gurdwara* is a Sikh temple; *mandir* is Hindu) in the United States.

● Turn left on 76th St. If you've been impressed with the places of worship so far, wait until you see what's on 46th Ave. Turn left for NYC's main Thai Buddhist temple. Go down its driveway to the shrines and statues, including a large reclining Buddha.

● Go back the way you came on 46th Ave., continuing to 74th St., where you turn right. Walk uphill for four blocks. Take a gander at the icons of St. Mary's Romanian Orthodox Church before turning right on Woodside Ave.

● Turn left on 75th St. On your right at 41st Ave., the United Sherpa Association has taken over the former St. Matthew's Lutheran Church and offers cultural events, social-services assistance, and Buddhist devotions for that Himalayan community. The tower you see ahead down 41st Ave. is a Chinese-speaking Seventh-Day Adventist church. Go one more block to Jackson Heights' transit hub at Broadway, where you can take the E, F, M, R, or 7 train.

POINTS OF INTEREST

Queens Center shopqueenscenter.org, 90-15 Queens Blvd., 718-592-3900

Ch'an Meditation Center chancenter.org, 90-56 Corona Ave., 718-592-6593

Sky Cafe 86-20 Whitney Ave., 718-651-9759

Himalaya Kitchen 86-08 Whitney Ave., 718-213-3789

Chao Thai 85-03 Whitney Ave., 718-424-4999

Moore Homestead Playground Broadway and 45th Ave.

ROUTE SUMMARY

1. Walk west on Queens Blvd. to Grand Ave., and cross over.
2. Walk on Broadway to Corona Ave., and turn right.
3. Go right onto 48th Ave. and continue around the high school until you're back on 48th.
4. Turn left on 92nd St.
5. Turn left on Corona Ave.
6. Turn right on 91st Pl.
7. Make a left on 43rd Ave., followed quickly by a right on Ithaca St.
8. Turn left on Whitney Ave.
9. Go through the park and turn right on 43rd Ave.
10. Merge onto Whitney Ave.
11. Turn right on Broadway, walking through Moore Homestead Playground along the way.
12. Bear left onto Woodside Ave.
13. Make a left on 76th St.
14. Turn left on 46th Ave.; at the Buddhist temple, turn around and head west.
15. Make a right on 74th St.
16. Go right on Woodside Ave., followed quickly by a left onto 75th St.

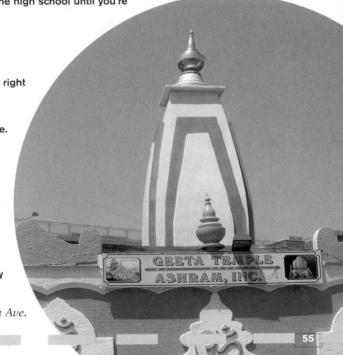

Hindu temple on Corona Ave.

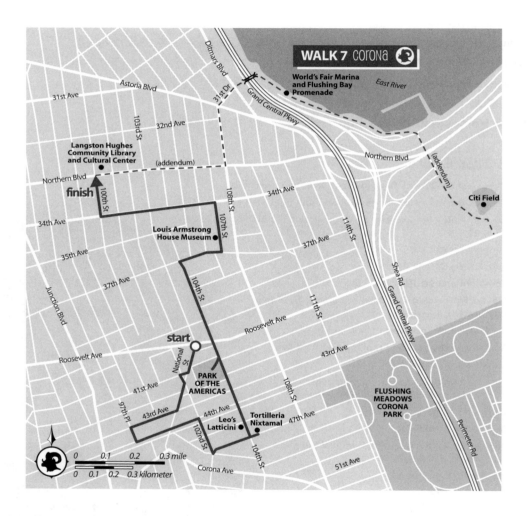

World's Fair Marina and Flushing Bay Promenade

East River

Dltmars Blvd

31st Dr

Grand Central Pkwy

Astoria Blvd

31st Ave

32nd Ave

103rd St

Langston Hughes Community Library and Cultural Center

(addendum)

Northern Blvd

Northern Blvd

(addendum)

Citi Field

finish

100th St

34th Ave

108th St

34th Ave

Louis Armstrong House Museum

107th St

37th Ave

111th St

Shea Rd

35th Ave

37th Ave

104th St

Junction Blvd

Roosevelt Ave

111th St

43rd Ave

Grand Central Pkwy

start

National St

Roosevelt Ave

PARK OF THE AMERICAS

108th St

FLUSHING MEADOWS CORONA PARK

41st Ave

43rd Ave

44th Ave

Leo's Latticini

Tortilleria Nixtamal

47th Ave

97th Pl

102nd St

104th St

51st Ave

Perimeter Rd

Corona Ave

0   0.1   0.2   0.3 mile

0   0.1   0.2   0.3 kilometer

7 corona: satchmo's wonderful world

BOUNDARIES: **Northern Blvd., 107th St., 47th Ave., 97th Pl.**
DISTANCE: **2.5 miles, plus optional 1.75-mile Flushing Bay Promenade extension**
SUBWAY: **7 to 103rd St.–Corona Plaza**

How did Corona become the crown jewel of Queens? Well, it isn't. Some say proud residents who thought it *was* a crown jewel proposed the name. Others say it came from Italian immigrants who moved in when the area was being developed by a company named Crown—*Corona* in Italian. Regardless of how the name originated, the neighborhood did deserve its own identity, as it had been called just West Flushing previously. Corona was served by the Long Island Rail Road until 1964, but the transit connection that made the biggest difference in its growth was the subway, which was extended to Corona via the elevated line now known as the 7 in 1917. Once predominantly Italian and Jewish, Corona today has the largest Latino population in the borough and has been represented in the State Assembly by Francisco Moya, the first Ecuadoran American ever elected to public office. This is the Corona that Paul Simon sings of ("Rosie, the queen of Corona") in "Me and Julio Down by the Schoolyard."

● Exit on the south side of Roosevelt Ave. to Corona Plaza, a public space created by its closure as a through street in 2012. Community events including a farmers' market and folkloric performances are held here. With the plaza on your left, walk on National St., named for a harness-racing track that was here in the 1850s and 1860s. It had a brief burst of popularity just as West Flushing was being mapped.

● Loop around the corner on your right at 41st Ave. to 102nd St. Look above the *iglesia*'s awning across 102nd, and you'll see that this Seventh-Day Adventist church occupies the former Corona Jewish Center, whose name is inscribed on the facade.

● Go left on 102nd St., then bear right as you pass between the two triangle parks so you're back on National St. The Spanish-speaking church on the right worships in the oldest building in Corona, erected for Union Evangelical Church around 1870. The Jehovah's Witnesses hall on the next block holds services in English, Spanish, Tagalog, and Twi—the latter two spoken by people from the Philippines and Ghana, respectively. And there's even more diversity right outside its doors, with a mosque adjacent and a Buddhist temple one block away. While this side epitomizes the present, across is a portrait of Corona past, as the storefronts on the other side have been here (albeit modified) since the late 1800s, when the nearby train station made this strip the center of town. Judging from its Second Empire style, the mansard-roofed house on the north corner of 43rd Ave. could date to the 1870s.

● Turn right on 43rd Ave. The beautiful firehouse on the left opened in 1913, while the FDNY was transitioning to a motorized fleet, and this was one of the first firehouses not built to accommodate horse-drawn fire engines.

● Make a left on 97th Pl. The new school on your right has taken the place of Tiffany Studios, where the famous lamps were produced from 1893 until the factory shut down during the Great Depression. The building was razed in 2013, and hundreds of shards of Tiffany glass were unearthed when the site was being cleared for the school.

● Turn left at 44th Ave. and walk beside the train tracks.

● Turn right on 102nd St.

● As you approach Nicolls Ave. to your right, make the first left, which is 47th Ave. Proceed to the green-shuttered white house on your left. Such country villas were quite common when it was built around 1871; now, however, it's very special, since it's the only such house that survives in the area. Known as the Edward E. Sanford House, after its first owner (it stayed in the family into the 1970s), it has been designated a city landmark. Cross 104th St. to Tortilleria Nixtamal, a restaurant that regularly makes best-Mexican-food-in-NYC lists. The secret is the *nixtamal,* a dried corn that the tortillas and tamales are made of. It's not corn flour but whole corn, and the restaurant prepares the nixtamal itself according to ancient Aztec tradition.

● Return to 104th St. and turn right. Another Corona eatery with a citywide reputation is on the left at 46th Ave., Leo's Latticini, maker of mozzarella and *bravissimi* sandwiches. How much of a local legend is this Italian deli? Its customers called the longtime owner Mama (hence the shop's alternate name), and since her death in 2009, the local elementary school and this block have been named in her honor.

On your right at 43rd Ave. stands the First United Methodist of Corona, as the church was known when it was erected in 1887 with a steeple that's now gone.

● Go into Park of the Americas at 41st Ave. You can see its earlier name, Linden Park, on the gateposts along with the images of linden leaves—they're also sculpted on the comfort station. Until 1947, the park contained a lake, also named Linden, but it was condemned due to pollution and filled in.

● Out of the park, continue north on 104th St. On your right at 37th Dr. stands Emanuel Lutheran, a congregation established in 1887 when Corona was heavily German, the language on its cornerstone at left. The streets around here are dominated by the massive steeple of Our Lady of Sorrows, another church founded in the early years of Corona. Take note of the church's handsomely carved wooden doors.

● Turn right in front of the church onto 37th Ave. The great jazz trumpeter Dizzy Gillespie lived in the apartment house on your near left at 106th St. from 1952 to 1966.

● Turn left on 107th St. and visit the house at #34-56 where Louis Armstrong resided for 28 years. Satchmo was already a world-renowned musician when he and his wife, Lucille, settled in this humble neighborhood shortly after marrying in 1943. He died at home in his sleep in 1971. Because the Armstrongs' home has been preserved—not re-created—with all their own furniture and personal belongings, their personalities and lifestyle really come alive for visitors. The couple splurged on interior decor: Wait until you see the bathroom with mirrored walls and the custom-designed kitchen finished in aquamarine lacquer! On the house tour, you get to hear Armstrong's voice singing and speaking, as he was an inveterate diarist both in writing and via reel-to-reel tape. Perhaps the nicest discovery of the tour is the superstar's deep connection to Corona: You can read his handwritten reflections and hear him discuss how his hit song "What a Wonderful World" reminds him of the neighborhood.

● Continue north on 107th St. to 34th Ave. and turn left. This last segment of the walk explores more of Corona's African American heritage, including Shaw African Methodist Episcopal Zion Church, a former synagogue at 100th St. (In the other direction on 34th Ave. are the Dorie Miller co-ops, a six-building complex between 112th and 114th Sts. that's been a primarily black middle-class community since opening in 1952. Its namesake was the first black recipient of the Navy Cross, and residents have included jazz musicians Cannonball Adderley, Nat Adderley, and Jimmy Heath.)

● Turn right on 100th St. and cross Northern Blvd. to the Langston Hughes Community Library and Cultural Center. Unique among Queens Library branches in that it began as a grassroots organization and was eventually incorporated into the public library system, the center is also the only place in NYC outside Manhattan that is designated a literary landmark by the American Library Association—see the plaque near the door. Go inside to view African and African American art and artifacts, including pieces that depict or were inspired by poet Hughes. The library also boasts the largest circulating collection of black-heritage reading material, and its research center contains the papers of Mary McLeod Bethune, Fannie Lou Hamer, and Countee Cullen.

● On 102nd St. south of Northern Blvd., board the Q23 bus back to the 7 train (0.6 mile away, if you want to walk). Or if you'd like to add a waterfront stroll, it's about 0.7 mile to the World's Fair Marina on Flushing Bay.

ADDENDUM

● From Northern Blvd., go left on 108th St., which turns into 31st Dr. across Astoria Blvd. Follow it onto the pedestrian bridge over the Grand Central Pkwy. The marina was developed for boaters to visit the 1964 World's Fair. It has 300 slips and winter storage, so boats are always docked there. A pleasant tree-lined promenade runs alongside the bay, and sculpted panels along its railing depict an animal and plant for every letter of the alphabet.

● Walk east (water on your left) until you reach two white, wavy fiberglass shelters— the Candela structures, the most neglected and most misunderstood fair relics. They resemble the shell-shaped buildings for which Spanish architect Félix Candela was renowned, but he designed neither them nor Mexico's pavilion at the fair (despite parks-department signage saying otherwise). During the fair, the structures had glass walls and housed exhibits and services of interest to marina users. A road behind the Candelas goes under the parkway, and from there you can walk through Citi Field's parking lot to the 7 at Mets–Willets Point.

POINTS OF INTEREST

Tortilleria Nixtamal tortillerianixtamal.com, 104-05 47th Ave., 718-699-2434

Leo's Latticini 46-02 104th St., 718-898-6069

Park of the Americas 104th St. and 42nd Ave.

Louis Armstrong House Museum louisarmstronghouse.org, 34-56 107th St., 718-478-8274

Langston Hughes Community Library and Cultural Center queenslibrary.org/branch
/langston-hughes, 100-01 Northern Blvd., 718-651-1100

aDDeNDUM POINTS OF INTErEST

World's Fair Marina and Flushing Bay Promenade Grand Central Pkwy. and 31st Dr.

rOUTe SUMMarY

1. Walk south on National St. from Corona Plaza.
2. Turn right on 41st Ave.
3. Turn left on 102nd St.
4. Bear right onto National St.
5. Turn right on 43rd Ave.
6. Turn left on 97th Pl.
7. Turn left on 44th Ave.
8. Turn right on 102nd St.
9. Turn left on 47th Ave.
10. Go north on 104th St. with a side trip into the Park of the Americas.
11. Make a right on 37th Ave.
12. Turn left on 107th St.
13. Make a left on 34th Ave.
14. Turn right on 100th St. and proceed to Northern Blvd.

aDDeNDUM

15. Turn left on 108th St.
16. Cross Astoria Blvd. and take 31st Dr. pedestrian bridge.
17. Make a right and walk along promenade.
18. Go right on road under the highway and continue through parking lot to 7 station.

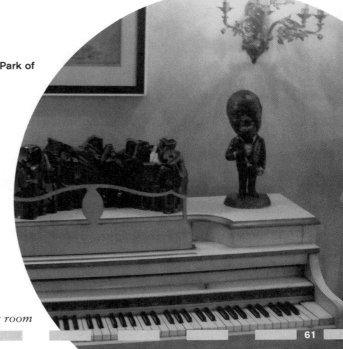

Inside Louis Armstrong's living room

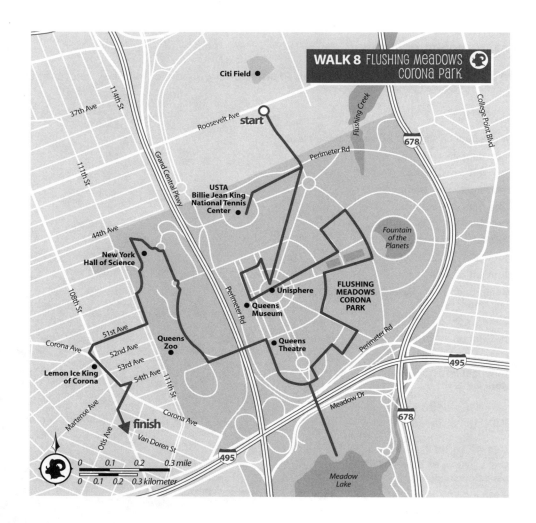

WALK 8 FLUSHING MEADOWS
CORONA PARK

Citi Field

37th Ave

114th St

111th St

Roosevelt Ave

start

Grand Central Pkwy

Perimeter Rd

Flushing Creek

College Point Blvd

678

USTA
Billie Jean King
National Tennis
Center

44th Ave

New York
Hall of Science

Fountain
of the
Planets

108th St

Perimeter Rd

Unisphere

FLUSHING
MEADOWS
CORONA
PARK

Queens
Museum

51st Ave

Corona Ave

52nd Ave

Queens
Zoo

53rd Ave

Queens
Theatre

Perimeter Rd

495

Lemon Ice King
of Corona

54th Ave

111th St

Martense Ave

Otis Ave

finish

Corona Ave

Van Doren St

Meadow Dr

678

495

Meadow
Lake

0   0.1   0.2   0.3 mile
0   0.1   0.2   0.3 kilometer

8 FLUSHING Meadows corona Park: Fair Play

BOUNDARIES: Roosevelt Ave., Fountain of the Planets, Meadow Lake, 108th St.
DISTANCE: Approximately 5 miles
SUBWAY: 7 to Mets–Willets Point

Sure, it possesses one of the more unfortunate place-names around, but Flushing Meadows has plenty of positive distinctions to make up for that. Flushing Meadows Corona Park, as it's known in full, has hosted two world's fairs. It's where the first papal Mass in the United States was celebrated, and where the United Nations General Assembly convened before UN permanent headquarters was completed. It's the venue for a Grand Slam tennis tournament and has been home field for both World Series and Super Bowl champions. It contains two museums and surpasses Manhattan's Central Park (and any other park in Queens) in size, offering nearly 900 acres of greenery and recreational options ranging from ice skating to miniature golf to model airplane flying. And the site's been immortalized in pop culture from *The Great Gatsby* to the Beastie Boys to *Iron Man 2*. This walk takes you all around Flushing Meadows, exploring world's fair relics both well known and hidden away, and concludes in Corona Heights, the neighborhood bordering the park to the west.

● Follow signs in the subway for the south side of Roosevelt Ave. and take the walkway into the park. This "Passerelle" served as the main entrance for the 1939 and 1964 World's Fairs. As you near the wavy-roofed structure, turn around to look at Citi Field, which replaced Shea Stadium in 2009. The New York Mets have been playing their home games at Flushing Meadows since Shea opened in 1964, and Shea was the home field of the NFL's New York Jets for two decades; it was also the locale for papal Masses in 1965 and 1979 and the first stadium to host a rock concert, when the Beatles famously played to 55,000 screaming fans. Shea was cavernous and rather ungainly, so Citi Field has been a great improvement; its facade and entry rotunda were modeled after Ebbets Field, the Brooklyn Dodgers' ballpark still mourned by many.

● Continue into Flushing Meadows. You get a preview of some of the fair remnants that you'll see from in-ground mosaics at David Dinkins Circle, named for the 1990–93 NYC mayor and tennis buff for his efforts to keep the US Open in Queens. The Open is played at the USTA Billie Jean King National Tennis Center, on your right. You're welcome to go in this public facility, which contains two stadiums and more than 40 indoor and outdoor courts.

● From Dinkins Circle, facing the sign about Dinkins, take the path on the right to the stainless steel Unisphere, the most recognizable icon of Queens. The disk-topped towers beyond it are the New York State Pavilion—built, like the Unisphere, for the 1964 World's Fair; you'll see those up close later. Proceeding counterclockwise as you face the Unisphere, make your first right, and walk toward *Freedom of the Human Spirit,* a bronze sculpture commissioned for the 1964 fair. Here, you can look into the tennis complex at Arthur Ashe Stadium; the Court of Champions, commemorating top Open players; and the *Soul in Flight* statue that honors humanitarian and onetime Open champ Ashe, the first African American tennis player to be ranked No. 1 in the world.

● Heading back toward the Unisphere, take winding Yitzhak Rabin Walk on your right through the America-Israel Friendship Grove. The state of Israel was in effect born at Flushing Meadows, as the 1947 UN vote to approve the partition of Palestine took place when the General Assembly met here. When you leave the grove on the other side, another world's fair sculpture, the abstract *Form,* is in front of you.

● Go to the left and walk to the Queens Museum, inside the only major building left from the 1939 World's Fair. It served as the New York City Pavilion during both fairs and as the UN General Assembly's meeting place from 1946 to 1951. It's now home to a must-see treasure, the Panorama of the City of New York. Created for the 1964 fair and updated since then, the Panorama is a detailed three-dimensional scale model of the city featuring buildings, bridges, and topographic features. The museum also displays fair memorabilia and a collection of Tiffany lamps, world-renowned objets d'art that came out of Queens (Tiffany's glassworks were located in Corona).

● From the museum, cross to the other side of Unisphere to the plaza where images of famous structures built for various world's fairs (the Eiffel Tower and Crystal Palace among them) are etched in the ground. Go down the steps and walk toward the *Rocket Thrower,* a symbol of space exploration, a major theme of the 1964 fair. Keep walking until you're between the two reflecting pools behind him, and then go on the pebble path on your left to the statue of George Washington.

Leave Washington via the path on *his* left, and when you reach pavement, make a right. This takes you to the Fountain of the Planets. Walk around it if you'd like— from the other side, you get the best sense of the park as fairgrounds—or just head back toward the Unisphere.

● Turn left once back at the *Rocket Thrower,* as if following his rocket's path. On your right stands the Column of Jerash, one of the oldest things you can find outdoors anywhere in New York. Dating to AD 120, this 30-foot-high marble column came from Jordan and stands on the site of that nation's 1964 pavilion.

● Continue in the direction you were going. Turn left at the next intersection, then make the second right. Within view and earshot of two busy highways, a Francis Bacon quote welcomes you to the Garden of Meditation, on your left. Feel free to use it as intended before you resume walking on the path.

● Make a right at the next intersection, followed quickly by a left. As you near the New York State Pavilion towers, you'll probably see skateboarders in the skate park created within a discontinued world's fair fountain. Behind it, under some trees, a semicircular sitting area (known as an exedra in Classical architecture) commemorates the park's papal connections.

● Take the nearby bridge that spans the Long Island Expy. to Ederle Terrace, overlooking Meadow Lake. In 1939, world's fair audiences enjoyed aquatic shows here featuring such swimming champs–turned–movie stars as Johnny Weissmuller and Esther Williams. You can follow a trail all the way around the lake, which

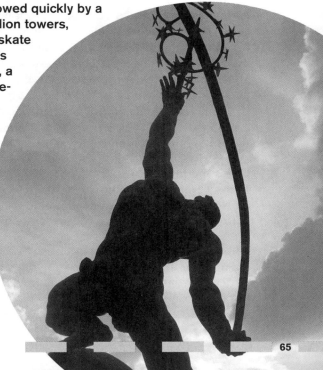

The Rocket Thrower *statue*

adds about 2.5 miles but affords an extraordinary experience: The brush and reeds in this wetlands provide a remote-feeling natural milieu uncharacteristic of NYC—though what's also unusual is being so immersed in nature while you are surrounded by highways, can see skyscrapers, and hear the whoosh of airplanes overhead! (LaGuardia Airport is just to the north.) If you go around the lake, you'll pass two dinosaur-themed playgrounds that pay homage to Sinclair Oil's popular Dinoland attraction of the world's fair. Both Meadow Lake and smaller Willow Lake south of it are fed naturally by Flushing River, also known as Flushing Creek, which flows from Flushing Meadows to the East River. If you're not up for the full walk, go partway and return to the terrace— or just enjoy the view from it. Then turn around and go back over the LIE bridge.

● Walk toward the New York State Pavilion—now's your chance to examine "America's Stonehenge" up close. Designed by Philip Johnson and unmistakably emblematic of the Space Age (they're real flying saucers according to *Men in Black,* whose climactic battle takes place here), the pavilion once featured elevators, an observation deck in its tallest tower, and a 166-foot-long terrazzo representation of New York State. Go to your left around the relic, watching out on the highway side for the time capsules buried during both world's fairs (not to be opened for an optimistic 5,000 years!). With the towers on your right, continue toward the Queens Theatre, ahead on your right. Mimicking the pavilion's silhouette, this renovated building was known during the fair as Theaterama, where a 360-degree scenic movie was screened inside and pop art by the likes of Andy Warhol and Roy Lichtenstein was exhibited on the exterior. Today a wide variety of theater, dance, and music is presented in its 470-seat theater and two smaller performance spaces.

● Cross the bridge to your left over the Grand Central Pkwy. Proceed straight ahead to the carousel, then turn right. You can go into the Queens Zoo, which focuses on North American animals, or settle for a glimpse into its petting zoo, on your left across from the dramatic bronze entry gates.

When you reach a fountain roundabout, a geodesic dome designed by Buckminster Fuller (now the zoo's aviary) is to your right, and another large, easily identifiable structure from the 1964–65 fair is to your left: the colored-glass-specked, undulating concrete sheets of the Great Hall. This building housed a science exhibit that grew into the New York Hall of Science, the museum of which it is now a part. Walk with it on your left and the tennis stadium visible to your right, and you'll end up at *Forms in Transit,* a rocketlike sculpture from the fair.

- Continue into the Hall of Science's parking lot and check out the Solar Walk along its sides, a series of globes indicating daylight and darkness around the world during the summer equinox (the smooth part of the globe is in daylight at the time on the clock next to it). As you walk toward the museum's entrance, you'll pass authentic NASA rockets, first put on display at the world's fair, and an aerospace-themed miniature golf course. All different branches of science are covered in exhibits and activities inside the museum.

- Exit the museum grounds and the park onto 111th St., and go left. Turn right on 51st Ave. and walk one block to 108th St. Corona Ave. crosses here too, forming the triangle where William F. Moore Park is situated. You're in Corona Heights, though probably only true old-timers would use that name; to everyone else, it's just part of Corona. Now largely Latino like the rest of Corona, this subneighborhood was once predominantly Italian American—filmmaker Martin Scorsese and college basketball coach Jim Valvano were both born in Corona. Remnants of that community include the bocce court here in what locals call Spaghetti Park and, across from the park at 52nd Ave., the Lemon Ice King of Corona, a Queens institution for decades before it was featured in the opening credits of *The King of Queens.*

- Proceed on 108th St., and across 53rd Ave., take the street to your left, which is Corona Ave. Make a left on 54th Ave. to see Congregation Tifereth Israel, the last synagogue in use in Corona. This wood-frame structure with Moorish windows and finial domes was restored for its centennial in 2011.

- Turn back in the direction you came from, but go on Otis Ave. to your left. Turn left on 108th St., and just before Van Doren St., look up on your right at the top of the apartment house at #55-22. We conclude our vicarious visit to the world's fairs with two of their lost but not forgotten symbols. That pointy object and the orb imprinted with 1939 on the roof represent the Trylon and Perisphere, icons of the 1939 fair. They were located where the Unisphere now stands and were scrapped for munitions during World War II.

Across 108th St., take the East Elmhurst–bound Q23 bus to the 103rd St.–Corona Plaza station of the 7.

POINTS OF INTEREST

Citi Field tinyurl.com/citifieldnyc, Roosevelt Ave. and 126th St., 718-507-8499

Flushing Meadows Corona Park Roosevelt Ave. and 114th St.

USTA Billie Jean King National Tennis Center tinyurl.com/bjktennis, Flushing Meadows Corona Park, 718-760-6200

Queens Museum queensmuseum.org, New York City Building, 718-592-9700

Queens Theatre queenstheatre.org, 14 United Nations Ave. S., 718-760-0064

Queens Zoo queenszoo.com, 53-51 111th St., 718-271-1500

New York Hall of Science nysci.org, 47-01 111th St., 718-699-0005

The Lemon Ice King of Corona thelemonicekingofcorona.com, 52-02 108th St., 718-699-5133

ROUTE SUMMARY

1. Go south from subway into park and take path on right from Dinkins Circle.
2. Go to right facing Unisphere, then make first right.
3. Reverse direction at Tennis Center gate, and walk through grove to your right.
4. Go left to Queens Museum. Proceed straight out of museum.
5. Turn left on pebble path, then right facing Washington statue.
6. Go right on pavement to Fountain of the Planets.
7. Head back toward *Rocket Thrower,* and turn left.
8. Make a left, then second right, then right at next intersection, then quick left.
9. Head south over bridge to Meadow Lake.
10. Go back across bridge and to your left around New York State Pavilion.
11. Go left at theater over bridge.
12. Turn right at carousel, continuing all the way to science museum.
13. Turn left on 111th St.
14. Make a right on 51st Ave., then head south on 108th St. from Moore Park.
15. Veer left onto Corona Ave., then turn left on 54th Ave.
16. Turn back and fork left onto Otis Ave. Go left on 108th St.

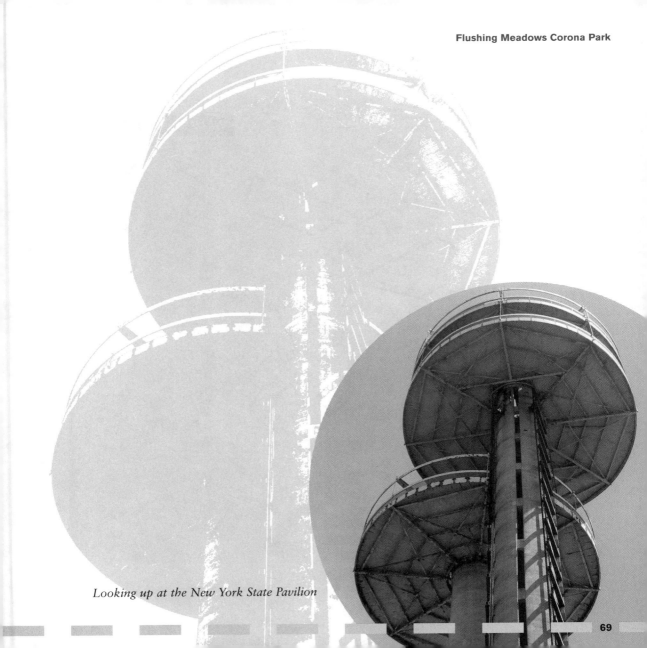

Looking up at the New York State Pavilion

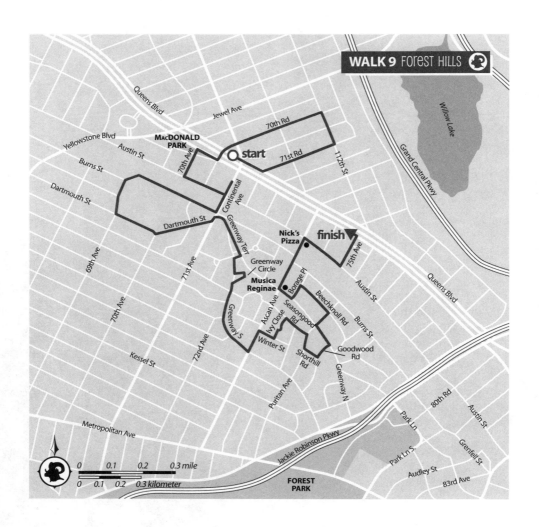

WALK 9 FOREST HILLS

Willow Lake

Queens Blvd

Jewel Ave

70th Rd

MacDONALD PARK

Yellowstone Blvd

Austin St

70th Ave

start

71st Rd

112th St

Grand Central Pkwy

Burns St

Dartmouth St

Continental Ave

Dartmouth St

Greenway Ter

Nick's Pizza

finish

75th Ave

69th Ave

71st Ave

Greenway Circle

Austin St

Queens Blvd

70th Ave

Musica Reginae

Borage Pl

Burns St

Ascan Ave

Beechknoll Rd

72nd Ave

Greenway S

Ivy Close

Seasongood Rd

Goodwood Rd

Kessel St

Winter St

Shorthill Rd

Greenway N

80th Rd

Austin St

Purtan Ave

Park Ln

Grenfell St

Metropolitan Ave

Park Ln S.

0   0.1   0.2   0.3 mile

0   0.1   0.2   0.3 kilometer

Jackie Robinson Pkwy

Audley St

83rd Ave

FOREST PARK

9 FOREST HILLS: BETTER HOMES AND GARDENS

BOUNDARIES: 69th Ave., 112th St., Goodwood Rd., Greenway S.
DISTANCE: 3.4 miles
SUBWAY: E, F, M, or R to Forest Hills–71st Ave.

Forest Hills started out as many Queens neighborhoods did: A developer buys up farmland, renames the area, and builds homes and infrastructure. It didn't end up like most neighborhoods, however. The developer sold part of the land, and a community was created, Forest Hills Gardens, that's one of the most desirable places to live in New York City. Inspired by England's garden city movement and modeled on its traditional villages, Forest Hills Gardens was designed with village greens, a central square, rich foliage, and beautiful houses. Even outside of the Gardens, Forest Hills boasts many nice houses and apartments as well as other advantages, such as a lively commercial district and express subway service. The first developer in Forest Hills was Cord Meyer, a company still headquartered on Queens Blvd., which laid out streets, set up utilities, and built hundreds of houses in what had been a township of six farms called Whitepot. "The Cord Meyer section" of Forest Hills generally applies to north of Queens Blvd. You go through just a bit of it at the beginning of this walk.

● Follow signs in the subway for 70th Rd. and 108th St., and exit on the north side of Queens Blvd. in front of a landmarked Art Deco bank. The businessmen who ran Ridgewood Savings wanted an auspicious structure for their first branch location and selected this triangular plot the bank could have to itself. Facing the bank, go to your right, and when you're at the front door, look up at the eagles sculpted into the semicircular roofline. Cross 108th St. and then 71st Ave. to an even older bank building, erected in the 1920s as a Masonic lodge. The diamond-shaped imprint above the sign used to hold the Masonic compass-and-square insignia.

● Continue past the bank and make a left on 71st Rd., in front of a supermarket that owes its Art Deco styling to the Carlton Terrace nightclub, which opened the building circa 1940 and remained a neighborhood hot spot into the 1970s.

● Turn left on 112th St. The synagogue on your right displays a plaque remembering the site's distinguished resident of 20 years, Helen Keller, the author, political activist, and advocate for the disabled. The first deaf and blind person to receive a college degree, Keller moved to then-rural Forest Hills in 1917 with Anne Sullivan, the "miracle worker" who'd taught her to communicate (dramatized in the play and movie of that name) and became a lifelong close friend. Sullivan's husband and Keller's secretary also lived in the house, and Sullivan died here in 1936.

- Cross 71st Ave. to First Presbyterian, the oldest church in Forest Hills and the one that Keller attended. The building was constructed in 1912 for the Forest Hills Free Church, later known as Union Church, which held nondenominational Protestant services because the neighborhood didn't have enough people to support separate churches—an idea innovative enough to warrant coverage in the *New York Times,* which called it "an experiment in practical Christianity which ought to be watched with interest by every small village the country over." Continuing to the end of the block, you see yet another house of worship, and it's quite a contrast with compact, old-fashioned First Presbyterian: Iglesia ni Cristo is typical of churches worldwide for this Filipino religion, in its size as well as in its spires and geometric patterns.

- Turn left on 70th Rd. and head back to Queens Blvd. Cross to the south side of the boulevard and make a right into MacDonald Park, which occupies a strip of land between traffic lanes. The park has hosted many civic gatherings over the years, from a 1964 campaign stop by US Senate candidate Robert F. Kennedy to a 9/11 candle-light vigil. Continue to the statue of the World War I veteran, a Forest Hills resident, for whom the park is named, and then on to the next circular area.

- Exit the park to your left, facing the post office. The WPA artwork created for the post office, instead of the usual mural inside, is an exterior sculpture titled *The Spirit of Communication;* some residents objected to the bare-breasted woman when it was unveiled in the late 1930s. The building's architect was Lorimer Rich, who'd come into prominence a few years earlier as codesigner of the Tomb of the Unknown Soldier at Arlington National Cemetery.

- Proceed on 70th Ave. On your left, the large building fronted by a multistory arched window and mosaic mural is a social and religious hub for Bukharians—Jews from Uzbekistan and other former Soviet republics in central Asia. At least three-quarters of the Bukharian Jews in the United States live in Queens, primarily Forest Hills and neighboring Rego Park and Kew Gardens. This building contains a synagogue, a school, an auditorium, the offices of a Bukharian newspaper, a senior center, and other facilities. Lev Leviev, an Israeli diamond mogul ranked among the world's richest people by *Forbes,* paid a significant portion of its $6 million cost, and his parents, Avner and Hana, are honored in the center's "official" Hebrew name, which you see to the left of the doors.

- Make a left on Austin St., lined with stores and restaurants. After passing two blocks of modern buildings, you can enjoy some of the original architecture of Forest Hills at 71st Ave. Across the avenue to your left, the half-timbered Tudor building is the neighborhood's earliest commercial site, erected circa 1911.

- Turn left and walk down 71st Ave., also known as Continental Ave., to the bishop's-crook lamppost. Look across at the large brick-and-terra-cotta building—a 1922 movie theater whose exterior, featuring heraldic ornamentation in both the blue and gold panels and the U-shaped band around them, has been preserved. Turn and head back in the direction from which you came. As you approach Austin St., admire the fast-food eatery across on the left—built as the Corn Exchange Bank in 1923. Note the crops sculpted in reliefs beside the windows.

- Continue underneath the railroad viaduct into Station Square, the picturesque entree to Forest Hills Gardens. In 1910 the Russell Sage Foundation, a philanthropy established by Olivia Sage with the inheritance from her financier husband, purchased 142 acres from Cord Meyer to create Forest Hills Gardens. It was supposed to be affordable to middle-income folks but quickly evolved into an affluent enclave. Here in Station Square in 1917, Theodore Roosevelt—the only native New Yorker to become president of the United States—headlined the Fourth of July festivities with a speech rallying support for the country's involvement in World War I. A couple of years earlier, the young community got a boost when the West Side Tennis Club, relocating from Manhattan, opened a new facility that would lure the US National Lawn Tennis Association championships from Newport, Rhode Island, to Forest Hills. The US Open was played here in the Gardens through 1977, as were 10 Davis Cup finals between 1914 and 1959.

- Make a right on Burns St. for the West Side Tennis Club (you'll have more time in Station Square later). On your left at Tennis Pl. is the Tudor-style clubhouse, built in 1913 to a design by Grosvenor Atterbury, the principal architect of Forest Hills Gardens. To see the stadium, continue on Burns St. and loop around the property via 69th Ave. and Dartmouth St. The first US stadium built specifically for tennis, it was also used for concerts, but they were discontinued in the 1980s because of complaints about noise and mess. A 2013 concert by Mumford & Sons kicked off the stadium's planned revival as a performance venue after it had been abandoned for more than a decade. The Beatles played here in 1964, arriving by helicopter from Manhattan; other legends to give concerts at Forest Hills include the Rolling Stones, Frank Sinatra, Jimi Hendrix, and Bob Dylan, who went electric for the second time (and was booed here too).

- At 70th Ave., note the different street signs—the city's standard green-and-white on one side of the avenue, Forest Hills Gardens' proprietary model (including a name, Herrick, for 70th Ave.) on the other side. The neighborhood also has its own unique lampposts. Make a left to continue on Dartmouth St. It won't take you long to get a feel for the extraordinary ambience of Forest Hills Gardens.

- Passing one of the community's private parks, turn left onto Continental Ave. and head back into Station Square. Now's your chance to explore this brick-paved show-place, including the pebble-faced Long Island Rail Road station. Towering above it all is the Forest Hills Inn, a hotel when it opened in 1912 and now a residential co-op. Enclosed walkways, which connect wings of the inn and the train station, bridge the streets radiating from the plaza. Once a center of social life for Forest Hills, the hotel offered indoor and outdoor dining, hosted community events and catered affairs, and contained a billiards room and squash court. A young piano player from Brooklyn by the name of Barry Manilow entertained in the lounge during its waning days.

- Beneath the tower, take Greenway Terr. out of Station Square. Peek inside the gates on your right at the late, lamented Tea Garden, then walk left of the village green to the Moorish-style church built in the 1930s by Christian Scientists. Cross to the other side of the green and continue on Greenway Terr. The house on your right at #65 was the longtime residence of Brooklyn-born actress Thelma Ritter, best remembered as Bette Davis's maid in *All About Eve* and James Stewart's nurse in *Rear Window.* Ritter was nominated for an Academy Award as Best Supporting Actress six times but never won, but she won the hearts of fellow Gardens residents as a friendly and involved neighbor. Go onto the green opposite her house. The tall eagle-topped pole is the mainmast from the yacht *Columbia,* two-time winner of the America's Cup under the co-ownership of J. P. Morgan. The rest of the boat was scrapped, while this mast was converted into a flagpole, dedicated by Theodore Roosevelt during his 1917 visit.

● Make a right on Greenway Cir. between the mast and the apartment complex at #150, which went up in the 1940s, replacing the Russell Sage Foundation offices.

● Cross Slocum Crescent and walk on Greenway S. Branch Rickey was living at #34 when, as general manager of the Brooklyn Dodgers, he made history by signing Jackie Robinson to a Major League contract. Rickey was active in the local church and gave away Dodgers tickets to its youth group. (Another famous resident of Forest Hills Gardens was Dale Carnegie, who was living at 27 Wendover Rd. when he wrote his mega-best-seller *How to Win Friends and Influence People.*)

● Turn left on Ascan Ave., then right on Winter St.

● Make a left on Ivy Close. Frederick Law Olmsted Jr., the landscape architect of Forest Hills Gardens, conceived the single-block roads like this as akin to parks and selected different plants for each one.

● Continue to wend your way through the Gardens with a right on Seasongood Rd., a right on Puritan Ave., a left on Shorthill Rd., and a left on Goodwood Rd.

● Turn left on Greenway N. The castle-like estate at #123 was the home of Trygve Lie while he served as first UN secretary-general. President

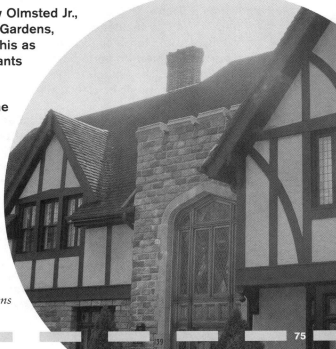

A home on Greenway N. in Forest Hills Gardens

Harry Truman may have visited him here. The United Nations convened at Flushing Meadows Corona Park in Queens during Lie's tenure, and in a farewell interview with *The New Yorker,* the Norwegian diplomat stated, "I am going to miss Granston Tower." He noted that his experience in Forest Hills disproved negative assumptions about New York, as his neighbors were always "gracious and cordial."

● Make a right on Puritan Ave.

● Turn left on Beechknoll Rd., walking alongside a village green once past Parkend Pl. On Borage Pl., #15 is the Community House, a home away from home for residents of the Gardens, who pay a membership fee to enjoy social activities, an indoor pool, and a gym. It has also run a nursery school and kindergarten since it opened in 1926–27.

● Turn left on Borage Pl., right on Greenway N., and right on Ascan Ave., bringing you in front of the Church-in-the-Gardens, whose appearance is as quaint as its name. The Grosvenor Atterbury–designed church features a tower crowned by a small iron spire known as a flèche. This building was dedicated in 1915, but the congregation was formed in 1912 by residents of five denominations, who decided to make it a Congregationalist church to be as inclusive as possible. For its centennial in 2012, church members re-created (in period dress) the first service in Station Square, where it had taken place. The church is the regular venue for Musica Reginae concerts, which feature chamber music or classically inspired world, jazz, and vocal music.

● Proceed on Ascan under the rail viaduct and out of Forest Hills Gardens. Nick's Pizza, on your right, is beloved for its thin-crust pizza, calzones, and cannoli. At Austin St., look at the street sign on the left designating the block Geraldine Ferraro Way. The trailblazing politician was living at 22 Deepdene Rd. in Forest Hills Gardens—her home for 35 years—when she ran for vice president in 1984, the first woman on a major-party presidential ticket. The sign is across from Our Lady Queen of Martyrs—the school here on Austin stands back-to-back with the church, which fronts Queens Blvd. Actor-comedian Ray Romano, who grew up in Forest Hills, attended Our Lady Queen of Martyrs School; so did David Caruso of *CSI: Miami* and Bob "Captain Kangaroo" Keeshan.

● Turn right on Austin St., which soon segues from commercial to residential. The first apartment house on your right, Tilden Arms, was named for tennis champ Bill Tilden after he'd won seven US Open titles (six consecutively) at Forest Hills in the 1920s.

MORE CELEBRITIES FROM FOREST HILLS

"The ultimate musical high school," *Rolling Stone* called Forest Hills High School in putting it on a list of US rock-and-roll landmarks that includes Graceland and the Motown studios. The school (at 110th St. and 67th Ave.) was cited for producing both the Ramones and Simon and Garfunkel, but its musical legacy is even more expansive: Burt Bacharach, the prolific Grammy- and Oscar-winning songwriter, also went to FHHS, as did the late opera star Tatiana Troyanos.

Television has also gotten its share of Forest Hills talent: Carroll O'Connor, who brought Queens into everybody's living room with his portrayal of Archie Bunker, grew up there, and it's the birthplace of Michael Landon and *The Simpsons'* Hank Azaria. But its biggest celebrity may be fictional: From the start of the Spider-Man comics, Peter Parker's hometown was identified as Forest Hills, Queens. Later issues gave his address as 20 Ingram St., an actual address in the Gardens.

Across 73rd Rd. on your left, the Holland House was promoted as having "all the advantages of a Park Avenue residence" when it opened in 1929 and has retained the prestige, evident in its elegant exterior and lobby, 24-hour doorman, and landscaped courtyard.

● Turn left on 75th Ave. These comely row houses on the right constitute Arbor Close, another of Forest Hills' urban-planning gems. They have a communal garden in the rear, and garages are lined up at the north end so that they don't disrupt the block's appearance. (Cord Meyer developed Arbor Close, on 75th Ave. and 75th Rd., and Forest Close, on 75th Rd. and 76th Ave., in the 1920s.)

● You reach Queens Blvd. beside a landmark firehouse, neo-Medieval in style rather than the neo-Georgian more common for firehouses of its era. The architecture has been described as "near-ecclesiastical," with its taller tower resembling one you'd see on a church. That tower, by the way, was designed for hose drying, the other tower for stairs.

There is an entrance to the 75th Ave. E and F subway station to your left as well as across Queens Blvd. (in front of Cord Meyer's offices).

POINTS OF INTEREST

MacDonald Park Queens Blvd. and 70th Ave.
Musica Reginae musicareginae.org, Church-in-the-Gardens, 50 Ascan Ave., 718-894-2178
Nick's Pizza 108-26 Ascan Ave., 718-263-1126

ROUTE SUMMARY

1. Walk east on Queens Blvd. to 71st Rd., and make a left.
2. Turn left on 112th St.
3. Go left on 70th Rd.
4. Cross Queens Blvd. and enter MacDonald Park.
5. Take 70th Ave. south away from the park.
6. Turn left on Austin St.
7. Make a left on 71st Ave., then turn around after viewing the old theater.
8. Turn right on Burns St.
9. Turn left on 69th Ave.
10. Turn left on Dartmouth St.
11. Make a left on Continental Ave.
12. Leave Station Square via Greenway Terr.
13. From the green, make a right on Greenway Cir., which becomes Greenway S.
14. Turn left on Ascan Ave.
15. Make a right on Winter St.
16. Turn left on Ivy Close.
17. Make a right on Seasongood Rd.
18. Turn right on Puritan Ave.
19. Go left on Shorthill Rd.
20. Turn left on Goodwood Rd.
21. Turn left on Greenway N.
22. Turn right on Puritan Ave.
23. Make a left on Beechknoll Rd.
24. Go left on Borage Pl.
25. Make a right on Greenway N.
26. Turn right on Ascan Ave.
27. Make a right on Austin St.
28. Go left on 75th Ave. to Queens Blvd.

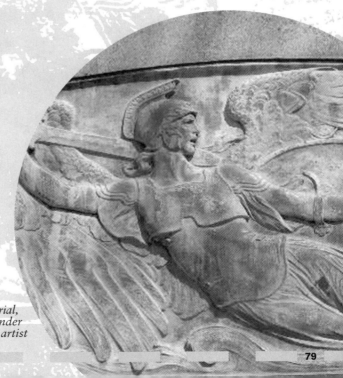

Forest Hills Gardens' World War I memorial, sculpted by local resident Adolph Alexander Weinman, a nationally known artist

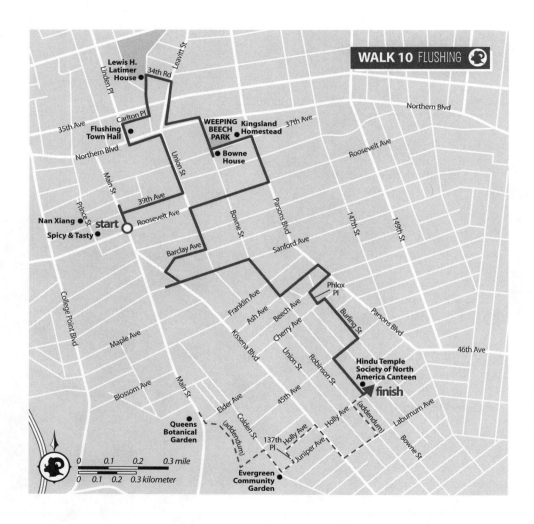

WALK 10 FLUSHING

Lewis H. Latimer House
34th Rd
Leavitt St
Linden Pl
35th Ave
Carlton Pl
Flushing Town Hall
WEEPING BEECH PARK
Kingsland Homestead
37th Ave
Northern Blvd
Northern Blvd
Union St
Bowne House
Main St
Prince St
39th Ave
Roosevelt Ave
Roosevelt Ave
Nan Xiang
start
Spicy & Tasty
Bowne St
Parsons Blvd
Sanford Ave
147th St
149th St
Barclay Ave
College Point Blvd
Maple Ave
Franklin Ave
Ash Ave
Beech Ave
Cherry Ave
Phlox Pl
Burling St
Parsons Blvd
46th Ave
Kissena Blvd
Union St
Robinson St
Hindu Temple Society of North America Canteen
finish
Blossom Ave
Main St
Elder Ave
Golden St
(addendum)
45th Ave
Holly Ave
Holly Ave
(addendum)
Laburnum Ave
Bowne St
Queens Botanical Garden
137th Pl
Holly Ave
Juniper Ave
Evergreen Community Garden
0   0.1   0.2   0.3 mile
0   0.1 0.2   0.3 kilometer

10 FLUSHING: STANDING UP FOR FREEDOM, STANDING OUT MULTICULTURALLY

BOUNDARIES: 34th Rd., Parsons Blvd., Holly or Laburnum Ave., Main St.
DISTANCE: 3.6 or 4.8 miles, depending on route chosen
SUBWAY: 7 to Main St.–Flushing

Within a single block of Bowne St. in Flushing are a synagogue, a Sikh temple, a Chinese Christian church, and a *mandir,* a Hindu house of worship. And why shouldn't there be? Flushing is, after all, the birthplace of religious freedom in America. One hundred and thirty years before the US Constitution was written, 30 of the village's most esteemed residents signed the Flushing Remonstrance, a 1657 letter to colonial governor Peter Stuyvesant opposing his religious intolerance. "Let every man stand and fall to his own master," they wrote, articulating a sentiment that would be codified in the First Amendment. John Bowne's house, where the document was composed, still stands, one of several exceptionally historic sights to be found amid the multicultural mélange of downtown Flushing. Known today as one of— very possibly the largest of—New York City's Chinatowns, Flushing has many Koreans and Indians too. More than two-thirds of the neighborhood's population is Asian, yet that's still just one facet of its far-reaching heritage.

● Exit at Roosevelt Ave. and walk north on Main St., toward the church steeple—which is practically brand-new, the previous one having been destroyed by a tornado in 2010. The church itself was erected in 1854, the third building for St. George's Episcopal, a congregation established in 1704. You can get more background from the Flushing Freedom Mile sign on the sidewalk (other historic sites also have such markers).

● Across Main St., the Chamber of Commerce building at #39-01 presents a nice Art Deco facade. Cross the street and walk east on 39th Ave., past Queens Crossing, an upscale "West meets East" shopping mall with event space and offices. An even larger mixed-use development is in the works beyond 138th St.: If built according to its $850 million plan, Flushing Commons will comprise residences, a small public park, and a YMCA along with commercial space. Hopefully, construction does not block your view to the left of Macedonia African Methodist Episcopal (AME) Church.

OTHER NEIGHBORHOODS OF FLUSHING

Murray Hill, which is east of downtown Flushing and has its own Long Island Rail Road stop, is named for the same family as Manhattan's Murray Hill (and the family that ultimately owned Kingsland Homestead). It contains a delightful Victorian home, Voelker Orth Museum, open to the public. The pink-and-white 1891 house has both flat and pitched roofs, an assortment of projecting bays and wings, eyebrow dormers, and a half-clapboard, half-shingled exterior—with the top-story shingles varying in shapes. Betty Voelker Orth's grandfather bought the house in 1899, and she lived in it her entire life (1926–1995). The grounds feature colorful flowering plants, an immaculate lawn, birdbaths, a grape arbor, beehives, and an herb garden. The Voelker Orth Museum is located at 38th Ave. and 149th Pl., just off hectic Northern Blvd.

On the other side of Northern Blvd., from 155th through 170th Sts., is **Broadway-Flushing.** Broadway *used* to be the name of Northern Blvd. in the area, and confusing though it may be, it's still the name of an LIRR stop. Broadway-Flushing was developed by Rickert-Finlay with covenants governing size and appearance of houses and yards that continue to be enforced by the homeowners' association. Thus it remains a verdant preserve of elegant Tudor, Colonial, and Arts and Crafts houses. A state and national historic district, Broadway-Flushing includes 11-acre Bowne Park (*below*), with a pond inhabited by turtles and bordered by two tall weeping willows.

The neighborhood west of Broadway-Flushing, **Linden Hill,** features a landmarked mansion at 145-15 Bayside Ave. **Queensboro Hill** is the part of south Flushing between Kissena Park and Queens College.

Among Flushing's religious groups, only the Quakers and Episcopalians organized earlier than Macedonia AME, which had two previous buildings at the same location. The church, founded in 1814, may have been a stop on the Underground Railroad.

● Turn left on Union St.

● At Northern Blvd., cross to the median and go left to the World War I monument, a female figure both powerful and poignant that resembles the Statue of Liberty but bears symbols of war and peace, a sword and laurel. Looking at her, you're also facing a National Guard armory (now used by the police department) built in 1905 on the site of the home where the Flushing Remonstrance was signed. Continue on the median past the trees. The ASPCA planter at the corner was placed here in 1909 as a water trough for horses. Cross to the western section of the mall: The obelisk is one of the nation's oldest Civil War memorials, dedicated in an 1866 ceremony attended by widows and orphans still in mourning.

● Use the crosswalk to go to the boulevard's south side and the wood-shingled Quaker meetinghouse. The Society of Friends held their first service here in November 1694, making it the oldest house of worship in New York. When Vlissingen (later Anglicized as Flushing) was settled in the mid-1600s, it was named for a Dutch city, though it was populated primarily by English, specifically Quakers fleeing the Puritan prejudice of New England. The street side is the back of the meetinghouse; if the gate's open, go into the true front yard. The cemetery there predates the building, as it was created in the 1670s on land that had been owned by John Bowne. A cast-iron stove from 1760 is inside the meetinghouse.

● Cross over to the north side of Northern Blvd. and Flushing Town Hall. You probably won't find any other building in the city that looks like this 1862 landmark, which is classified as early Romanesque in style. Flushing was an independent town, and Queens not yet part of NYC, when the building opened with municipal offices downstairs and a great hall for social and civic events upstairs. It is now a cultural center. In admiring the nifty features higher up on the building, don't overlook its beautifully detailed portico. Inside, the gift shop showcases crafts and other products made by Queens-based artisans.

● Walk north on Linden Pl.

- Turn right on Carlton Pl., where the last prewar holdouts in the area are clustered.

- Make a left on Leavitt St. and go two blocks to the landmarked home of Lewis H. Latimer, an African American inventor who provided invaluable assistance to both Alexander Graham Bell and Thomas Edison. The Massachusetts-born son of escaped slaves, Latimer was a self-taught draftsman who did the drawings submitted by Bell in his patent application for the telephone and was Edison's chief draftsman and patent expert. Latimer's own patents included the carbon filaments used in lightbulbs. In this home, Latimer pursued his hobbies of painting and poetry and hosted the likes of Paul Robeson and W. E. B. Du Bois.

- Turn right on 34th Rd.

- Make another right on Union St.

- Turn left on Northern Blvd. in front of Flushing High School. This campus for NYC's oldest public high school was designed to evoke such august seats of learning as Oxford and Cambridge. Nonetheless, the gargoyles steal the show.

- Turn right on Bowne St. In front of the Cambridge Court apartments, on your right, a large rock marks the spot where George Fox, the Englishman who founded Quakerism, preached outdoors in 1672 on the farm of John Bowne, whose house still stands at the 37th Ave. intersection. Cross over to the Bowne House, the oldest structure in Queens. Before the Friends meetinghouse was built, John Bowne hosted Quaker services in this home, in open defiance of Peter Stuyvesant's prohibition of all religions other than Dutch Reformed. Subsequent generations of Bownes left their mark too—in the shipping and publishing industries, as antislavery and education advocates, and in politics (Walter Bowne was mayor of New York in the 1830s). They were also joined through marriage to the Parsons family; nine generations of the Bowne and Parsons family lived in the house before it was turned into a museum.

- Behind the Bowne House, walk through the Margaret I. Carman Green and make a left into Weeping Beech Park. It occupies land that was part of the Parsons nursery, which introduced hundreds of plant species to the United States, including the Japanese maple and pink dogwood, and was the first commercial grower of rhododendrons and azaleas. It carried on a Flushing tradition that started with the Prince nursery, the first US commercial nursery (established in 1737). Make the first right to see an homage to Flushing's horticultural heritage in the spray-shower area: the names and leaves of various tree species imprinted in cement. You also have a good view of Kingsland Homestead, built circa 1785, on the other side of the fence.

● Leave the playground where you entered, and make a left on 37th Ave. Then go left onto the Kingsland grounds. The house was built for Charles Doughty but got its name from his son-in-law Captain Joseph King, its second owner. Inside, the oldest items are a set of china King brought back from England and a Federal-style mahogany bookcase, both from around 1800. The house also features a parlor filled with Victorian-era furnishings and "Aunt Mary's Closet," a display case of assorted possessions—doll clothes, travel souvenirs, and a notebook, among them—of Mary Murray, King's granddaughter, who lived here into her 70s and kept a diary that's provided a lot of historical information about the home. The Queens Historical Society, based at Kingsland, maintains the home and sponsors themed exhibitions. On the east side of the property is a group of weeping beech trees, the offspring of the original weeping beech that Samuel Bowne Parsons planted in 1847 from a shoot he'd acquired in Belgium. All US weeping beeches probably spawned from that tree, which grew to more than 60 feet tall with a 14-foot-wide trunk.

● Continue on 37th Ave. to Parsons Blvd., and turn right. This second half of the walk focuses on present-day Flushing's multiculturalism—John Bowne's legacy, you might say. Your first example lies south of 38th Ave., with a Conservative synagogue across from the Sikh Center.

● Turn right on Roosevelt Ave. The Bowne Street Community Church, at the end of the block, was completed in 1892 for a Dutch Reformed congregation established in the 1840s. About a decade into that congregation's existence, a group of parishioners split off to form a Congregationalist church. With the changing population in the 1970s, both churches' memberships dwindled and the two organizations ultimately reunited. The sanctuary contains Tiffany stained glass windows. After you cross Bowne St., stay on the right so you can read an oft-overlooked plaque on the westernmost wall of the grocery store about Daniel Carter Beard, for whom the landscaped mall on Northern Blvd. is named.

- Turn left on Union St. If you look up at the firehouse's doorway (beneath the companies' names), you'll see angels that are part of a 9/11 memorial mural, which you can see in its entirety if the door is closed. Continue over the railroad tracks and across 41st Ave., where St. Michael's makes a good case for modern religious architecture in a neighborhood filled with historic houses of worship. The church does have a long history—going back more than a century and a half—but this complex, with both red tile and copper roofs, is its third home.

- Go right on Barclay Ave. Symbols of the Apostles are carved into the church facade on this side.

- Turn left on Kissena Blvd. Positioned at an angle atop a long staircase at the next intersection is the Free Synagogue of Flushing. Its neoclassical building, which is listed on the National Register of Historic Places, bears a quotation from the Book of Isaiah above its Corinthian columns. Note also the sculptings in the door pediments.

- Turn right on Sanford Ave. so you can see more of this majestic building, including its copper dome and stained glass windows made in Europe. The white mansion next door has been attributed to architect Stanford White and predates the Civil War.

- Reverse direction and head east on Sanford Ave. Opposite the park at Union St., First Baptist Church's building represents the Flushing of the late 19th century, its multilingual signage the Flushing of the 21st century.

- Turn right on Bowne St. To the left at Franklin Ave., you can't miss the Korean American Presbyterian Church of Queens, a bilingual megachurch. South of Franklin, you've entered Waldheim, a wealthy subdivision developed after 1875. The name is German for "house in the woods," which is what the developers aimed for, building 70 or so large, individualistic houses on spacious, leafy lots along landscaped streets. The Waldheim name fell out of favor due to anti-German sentiment during World War I, but residents and preservationists have been fighting for the neighborhood ever since the first apartment building went up within its borders in the 1920s. By now, as much has been demolished or significantly altered as preserved, but interesting old houses do remain, including one on your left as you reach Ash Ave.

● Turn left on Ash Ave. The first two properties on each side illustrate exactly what people have been striving to save—and to prevent. You will continue to see turn-of-the-century mini-mansions alternating with aesthetically inferior newer housing as you walk the streets of old Waldheim. Their curved rather than right-angle corners were part of its design.

● Turn right on Parsons Blvd. Nichiren Shoshu, a branch of Buddhism begun in 13th-century Japan, is practiced in the modernistic structure on the right, which is unusually plain for a Buddhist temple.

● Make a right on Beech Ave. In keeping with the woodsy theme of Waldheim, and in tribute to the pioneering nurseries of Flushing, most roads in this part of town are named for trees and plants.

● Turn left on Phlox Pl. and left on Cherry Ave. Next to a picturesque if careworn early-1900s house is the Won Buddhist Temple.

● Turn right on Burling St. Won is a Korean denomination of Buddhism, and here's where you see the front of the temple, including its adorned mailbox. A few of Waldheim's original houses survive on this block. To your left is Flushing Hospital, the oldest in Queens.

● Make a right on 45th Ave., formerly Forest Ave.

● Turn left on Bowne St. The Asa-mai temple in the house at #45-32 is for Hindus from Afghanistan. A temple in the South Indian style is farther down the block, and no tour of the

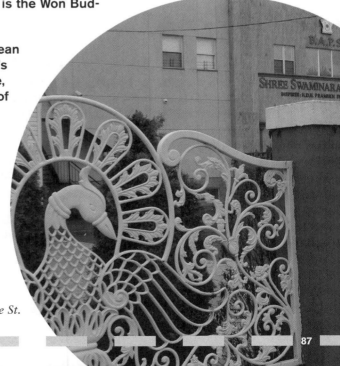

Entrance to a Hindu temple on Bowne St.

cultural diversity of Flushing would be complete without this pièce de resistance, the so-called Ganesha Temple. Run by the Hindu Temple Society of North America, it's perhaps the most grandiose Hindu place of worship in the West. Before this temple was built, the society occupied a former church on the site—the services held there in 1970 are believed to be the first public Hindu worship services ever held in the United States. The temple was designed in accordance with the Agama Shastras scriptures and constructed mostly of imported materials. You should take off your shoes and enter, going into both the main altar-filled room (to your left upon entering) and the ornate open-air wing (to the right). You're also welcome to dine at the Canteen, the temple's cafeteria, which has no frills but lots of fans from both in and outside the temple community. Its tasty, reasonably priced South Indian menu is led by *dosas,* filled crepes made from a rice-and-lentil batter. Entrance to the Canteen and gift shop is on Holly Ave. Afterward, you can wait on the same side of Holly west of Bowne St. for the Q27 bus back to the Main St. subway. Or if you're up for more walking and you'd like to see a green side of Flushing, continue.

ADDENDUM

- Walk west on Holly Ave. and make a left on Robinson St., where you'll find another Hindu temple, this one dedicated to the teachings of Shri Shirdi Saibaba and completed in 2010. Anywhere else in the United States, this would be a large Hindu temple, but compared with its Ganesha neighbor, it seems midsize.

- Make a right on Laburnum Ave.

- Turn right on Kissena Blvd. An elaborate Buddhist temple is on your left at the next corner.

- Turn left on Holly Ave., beside yet another big Hindu temple. Around the corner from the Hindu Center (on Geranium Ave.) is the Muslim Center of New York; you may be able to see its minaret from Holly Ave.

- Go left on 137th Pl.

- Make a right on Juniper Ave.

- At Colden St., cross to the other side for the entrance to massive Evergreen Community Garden, which has about 300 plots on more than 5 acres. As long as you're here when it's open, you're welcome to wander around its tidy plots of flowers and produce, which includes many vegetables used in Korean cuisine.

- Back on Colden St., continue north. Opposite Geranium Ave., turn left onto the blacktop path between playgrounds. Make a right on the far side of Silent Springs Playground, walking on the grass next to the basketball courts and then onto a dirt path. Pass the baseball and cricket fields, then go right at a paved path. This is all the western section of Kissena Corridor Park, which links Flushing Meadows Corona Park with Kissena Park; another Kissena Corridor on Kissena Park's east side connects to Cunningham Park, which is connected to Alley Pond Park by the Long Island Motor Pkwy. walking and biking trail—altogether they form a 6-mile greenbelt across Queens.

- Cross Main St. upon leaving the park, and go to the right. At the next intersection, enter the Queens Botanical Garden, which originated as an exhibit at the 1939 World's Fair and is now eight times larger. In addition to many plant varieties, it features botanical models of ecological sustainability and conservation and hosts programs geared to the ethnic communities of Flushing.

- Depending on where you exit the garden, take the northbound Q44 or Q20 on Main St. or Q58 on College Point Blvd. to the Main St. 7. Dining recommendations near the subway include Prince St., one block west of Main St. It has a great selection of Asian eateries between Roosevelt and 37th Aves.; standouts include Spicy & Tasty, a Szechuan restaurant with a citywide reputation, and Nan Xiang for its soup dumplings (*xiao long bao*).

POINTS OF INTEREST

Flushing Town Hall flushingtownhall.org, 137-35 Northern Blvd., 718-463-7700

Lewis H. Latimer House tinyurl.com/latimerhouse, 34-41 137th St., 718-961-8585

Bowne House bownehouse.org, 37-01 Bowne St., 718-359-0528

Kingsland Homestead queenshistoricalsociety.org, 145-35 37th Ave., 718-939-0647

Hindu Temple Society of North America Canteen nyganeshtemple.org/canteen, 143-09 Holly Ave., 718-460-8493

Spicy & Tasty spicyandtasty.com, 39-07 Prince St., 718-359-1601

Nan Xiang 38-12 Prince St., 718-321-3838

aDDenDum Points of Interest

Evergreen Community Garden Colden St. at Juniper Ave.

Queens Botanical Garden queensbotanical.org, 43-50 Main St., 718-886-3800

route summary

1. Walk north on Main St. from Roosevelt Ave.
2. Go east on 39th Ave.
3. Turn left on Union St.
4. Walk west on Northern Blvd. median.
5. Cross to the south and then north side of Northern Blvd.
6. Head north on Linden Pl., turning right onto Carlton Pl.
7. Turn left on Leavitt St. and right on 34th Rd.
8. Make a right on Union St.
9. Turn left on Northern Blvd.
10. Make a right on Bowne St.
11. Go through Carman Green, into Weeping Beech Park, then left onto 37th Ave.
12. Turn right on Parsons Blvd.
13. Make a right on Roosevelt Ave.
14. Make a left on Union St.
15. Turn right on Barclay Ave.
16. Make a left on Kissena Blvd.
17. Go right on Sanford Ave., then turn around and head east.
18. Turn right on Bowne St.
19. Make a left on Ash Ave.
20. Turn right on Parsons Blvd.

21. Make a right on Beech Ave., a left on Phlox Pl., and another left on Cherry Ave.
22. Make a right on Burling St.
23. Go right on 45th Ave.
24. Turn left on Bowne St.
25. Make a left on—or walk through Ganesha Temple to—Holly Ave.

ADDENDUM

26. Go west on Holly Ave. to Robinson St., and turn left.
27. Turn right on Laburnum Ave., then right on Kissena Blvd.
28. Turn left on Holly Ave.
29. Make a left on 137th Pl. and a right on Juniper Ave.
30. Turn right on Colden St.
31. Walk through Kissena Corridor Park.
32. Go right on Main St. to botanical garden.

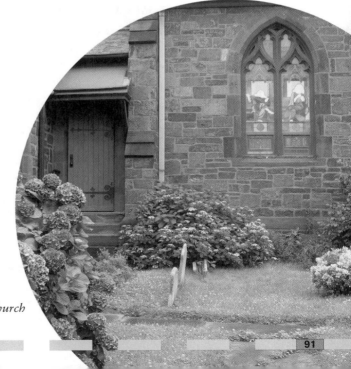

One corner of St. George's Episcopal Church

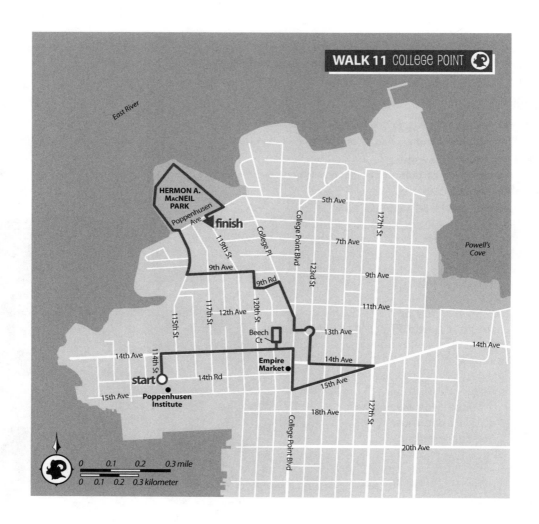

WALK 11 COLLEGE POINT

East River

HERMON A.
MacNEIL
PARK

Poppenhusen Ave

finish

5th Ave

College Point Blvd

123rd St

127th St

Powell's Cove

7th Ave

119th St

College Pl

9th Ave

9th Ave

9th Rd

9th Ave

11th Ave

115th St

117th St

12th Ave

120th St

Beech
Ct

13th Ave

14th Ave

14th Ave

14th Ave

start

114th St

Empire
Market

14th Ave

14th Rd

15th Ave

15th Ave

Poppenhusen
Institute

18th Ave

127th St

College Point Blvd

20th Ave

0   0.1   0.2   0.3 mile
0   0.1   0.2   0.3 kilometer

11 COLLEGE POINT: rubber-made

BOUNDARIES: MacNeil Park, 127th St, 15th Ave., 114th St.
DISTANCE: 2.7 miles
SUBWAY: 7 to Main St.–Flushing, transfer to Q65 bus

St. Paul's College had virtually no impact on College Point aside from inspiring its name. The seminary existed for only about 15 years, and its buildings were eventually demolished. If College Point's name were to reflect the biggest influence in its development, it would probably be called Poppenhusen—as in Conrad Poppenhusen, the German-born industrialist who ran a rubber-goods factory there in the 19th century and gave the town a bank, a church, a railroad, paved streets, schools, and housing where his employees lived. College Point has had other identities besides Poppenhusen's factory town, among them a German American stronghold (*Freie Presse* was a locally published newspaper) and recreational hot spot. Thanks to its waterfront location, College Point was a popular destination for day trips and weekend getaways, offering accommodations from bathhouses to full-fledged resorts for all types of fun seekers, who enjoyed beer gardens, picnic parks, beaches, and sporting grounds. Today, a city park takes full advantage of College Point's perch on the north shore of Queens.

● Get off the bus on 14th Rd. at 114th St., across the street from the Poppenhusen Institute. Conrad Poppenhusen established the first free kindergarten in the United States, along with a vocational secondary school, in this building, and at its grand opening in May 1870 he explained that his duty as an employer "could best be fulfilled by giving to your children the means of a better education." The institute has always sought to uphold that mission over the years, offering such training as welding classes for women during World War II and English-language lessons for immigrants. Poppenhusen created the institute as both a civic and educational center: It housed a public library, a bank, and the village hall. It still functions as a community center—hosting music and martial arts classes, concerts and plays, and special events—and owns a treasure trove of artifacts. The splendid ballroom is available for event rental and has made appearances on the TV series *Boardwalk Empire.* Go inside if the building's open, and walk around it outdoors.

POPPENHUSEN PLUS: MANUFACTURING IN COLLEGE POINT

While College Point still has an industrial sector, manufacturing has decreased from the time when it had multiple textile mills, metalworks, and breweries. The community's leading industrialist, Conrad Poppenhusen, held the exclusive rights to Charles Goodyear's vulcanizing process, but he wasn't the only rubber-goods manufacturer in town. Kleinert, inventor of the shower cap and shower curtain, was also based in College Point, and its name is visible on its former factory on 127th St. at 20th Ave. Still in business out of state, Kleinert specialized in apparel-related products like rubber pants for babies, which were worn over cloth diapers.

A couple of blocks from the Poppenhusen Institute, the three-story brick building that stretches from 15th Ave. to 14th Rd. on 110th St. was built for the Chilton paint company, which made the signature black lacquer for Steinway & Sons pianos, manufactured just across Flushing Bay in Astoria. Chilton took over the site from a sawmill, and the classic house with a mansard roof across from it on 14th Rd. was built for the mill owner.

The aviation industry also thrived in College Point: It had three airplane manufacturers and a commercial airfield. Flushing Airport opened in 1927 and was the city's busiest airport before LaGuardia opened 12 years later. It continued to be used by private planes until it shut down in the mid-1980s. The untended property has turned into wetlands, while College Point Corporate Park was developed around it. The NYPD has just constructed a 30-acre, $660 million Police Academy campus at the College Point Corporate Park, which also includes a *New York Times* printing plant, a shopping mall with a multiplex, and other commercial and industrial tenants.

- Walk north on 114th St., away from the Poppenhusen Institute and Flushing Bay. On your right, past four close-together houses, the brick building with a bay window over its garage was a firehouse at the turn of the century.

- Make a right on 14th Ave. The commercial complex on your left occupies the site, extending to the river, of Donnelly's, which was College Point's second-largest resort. The 27-acre property, which had ball fields, a dancing pavilion, bowling alleys, and shooting galleries, welcomed business and political groups in addition to leisure travelers. One such gathering in the early 1880s launched the political career of Theodore Roosevelt, who announced his candidacy for the New York State Assembly at Donnelly's. Proceeding along the avenue, you see a steeple up ahead, and after 118th St., you're in front of the charming clapboard church to which it belongs. Poppenhusen bankrolled construction of First Reformed in the 1870s. Read the sign on the iron fence in front. A block down 119th St. to your right was Flessel's, a German restaurant that opened in the early 1870s and, amazingly, survived until 1998, the last of College Point's beer gardens.

- Opposite 121st St., turn left into Beech Ct., noting the stone gateposts (behind the DEAD END signs). Nine houses are arrayed around a central lawn on the former estate of Herman Funke, who owned a local silk mill. Walk around the court and return to 14th Avenue.

- Make a left back onto 14th Ave. At the corner on your left, this branch of the Queens Library exists courtesy of two philanthropic millionaires—and a lot of regular Joes. The 1904 building was paid for by Andrew Carnegie, out of his $5.2 million bequest to the city for a network of libraries, and its first 3,200 books came from Poppenhusen Institute. The people of College Point purchased the land for it by donating money, including $1 from each employee of the Poppenhusen factory. For this branch alone among his 65 endowed libraries, Carnegie hired the prestigious architecture firm of Heins & Lafarge, who'd designed parts of the Cathedral of St. John the Divine and the Bronx Zoo. Its highly ornamented entryway includes open books sculpted above the lamps.

- Turn right on College Point Blvd.—caught halfway between generic commercial strip of the 21st century and small-town main street of yesteryear. Empire Market, at #14-26, provides the neighborhood's last taste of the old world: Open since 1921, it's the only German-food purveyor left. You may never have seen such an extensive menu of sausages, cold cuts, and smoked meats as that made by the Lepines, the family who's run the shop for three generations. They prepare them in their own smokehouse on the premises. Back on the boulevard, you can spot some buildings from long ago as you walk. See, for example, above ground level at #14-17 and #14-54.

- Turn left on 15th Ave. The dominant presence around 123rd and 124th Sts. is St. Fidelis, the oldest Catholic congregation in College Point, organized in 1856 by an Austrian-born priest (who's buried on the property). On your right at 126th St. is a truly remarkable survivor, all the way from 1868: Farrington's, which has been a service station since horses, not cars, got serviced—and has been owned by the same family all that time.

- Make a sharp left onto 14th Ave. at 127th St., an intersection known as Five Corners. A German restaurant in the half-timbered building on 14th Ave. stayed in business until 2009. The building with a conical tower on the left corner of 124th St. is a convent for nuns who teach at St. Agnes, a girls' high school, and is older than the St. Fidelis church, which dates to 1894.

- Turn right on 123rd St. Next to the parking lot on the left stands a Queen Anne–style meetinghouse that's listed on the National Register of Historic Places. Known as Firemen's Hall, it was erected in 1906 for a volunteer fire company but more recently has been a senior center and Little League headquarters. On your right, the house at #13-17 dates to the 1850s, with obvious modifications. The taller house next to it is also 19th-century, built for the owner of a silk mill. And then, a couple of doors away, there's an antebellum mansion . . . in the middle of the street. The house was here first—built in 1857 on the 14-acre estate of dry-goods merchant Herman A. Schleicher—and the roads were routed around it when a street grid was introduced decades later. Go to your right, walking around to its front facing 13th Ave. Its porch was not enclosed originally, and the house was positioned facing west to catch sea breezes and sunsets.

- With the house behind you, go one block on 13th Ave. and make a right on College Point Blvd. Another block farther and you're face-to-face with Conrad Poppenhusen, honored with a bronze bust for which College Point residents raised funds the year after his death. Poppenhusen's house stood to your left, and he deeded this lot to the public for parkland (a larger park named for him, also on land he once owned, is off 20th Ave.).

- Walk on the left side of the triangle, which is College Pl. As you pass some big old houses, remember that this was the ritzier north side of town, where factory owners and managers lived.

- Make a left on 9th Rd., between two stone pillars.

- Turn right on 120th St.

● Turn left on 9th Ave. You'll see some nicer-looking, generally older houses closer to the water.

● Make a right to head north on 115th St. Edgewater Estates to your left was designed with the area's ever-increasing Asian population in mind: Note that this section is on Dalian Ct.—named, like the development's other "street," Taipei Ct. (a block south), for a city in China.

● At the end of 115th St., cross Poppenhusen Ave. to MacNeil Park, a hidden gem. Tucked away at one of the northernmost points of Queens, 3 miles from the nearest subway, the park is little-known outside the neighborhood despite having possibly the best views of anywhere in the city.

Go to your left onto the riverside path. At or near the stairs, ascend the bluff into the park and make a left on the path. Then go onto the lawn, toward the sign about the Living Memorial Grove, which was planted in this park because of its view of the World Trade Center. This park occupies the site of the short-lived St. Paul's College. It's remembered more, however, as the location of a mansion, originally owned by William Chisolm, that stood here from the 1840s up to 1941 and was used by Mayor Fiorello LaGuardia as a summer city hall. Some old-timers still refer to the park as Chisolm's. The park's namesake, Hermon A. MacNeil, was a nationally known sculptor who lived in College Point. His NYC work includes a George Washington statue in Greenwich Village's Washington Square Park and a war memorial on Northern Blvd. in Flushing.

● Outside the park entrance on 119th St., take the Q25 to the Flushing 7.

POINTS OF INTEREST

Poppenhusen Institute poppenhuseninstitute.org, 114-04 14th Rd., 718-358-0067
Empire Market empire-market.com, 14-26 College Point Blvd., 718-359-0209
Hermon A. MacNeil Park Poppenhusen Ave. and 115th St.

route summary

1.   Walk north on 114th St. from 14th Rd.

2.   Turn right on 14th Ave.

3.   Go in and out of Beech Ct., then go left on 14th Ave.

4.   Make a right on College Point Blvd.

5.   Turn left on 15th Ave.

6.   Make a left onto 14th Ave. at 127th St.

7.   Make a right on 123rd St.

8.   From the Schleicher mansion, head west on 13th Ave.

9.   Turn right onto College Point Blvd.

10.   Go left onto College Pl.

11.   Make a left on 9th Rd.

12.   Turn right on 120th St.

13.   Make a left on 9th Ave.

14.   Go right on 115th St. to the park at Poppenhusen Ave.

15.   After walking in MacNeil Park, return to Poppenhusen Ave. at 119th St.

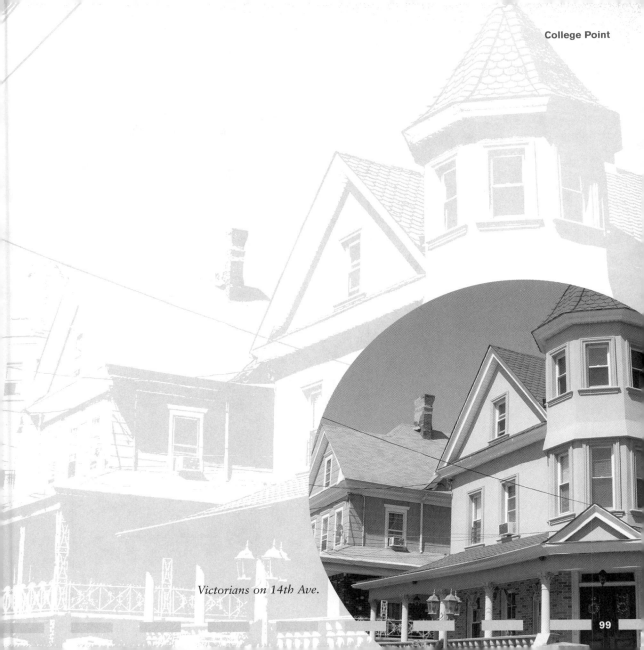

Victorians on 14th Ave.

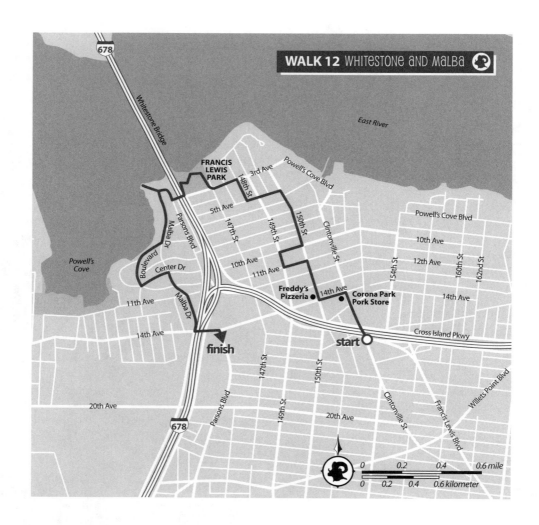

WALK 12 WHITESTONE AND MALBA

678

Whitestone Bridge

East River

FRANCIS LEWIS PARK

3rd Ave

Powell's Cove Blvd

148th St

5th Ave

Powell's Cove Blvd

10th Ave

12th Ave

154th St

160th St

162nd St

147th St

149th St

150th St

Clintonville St

Parsons Blvd

Malba Dr

Powell's Cove

Boulevard

Center Dr

10th Ave

11th Ave

14th Ave

Malba Dr

11th Ave

Freddy's Pizzeria

14th Ave

Corona Park Pork Store

14th Ave

14th Ave

finish

start

Cross Island Pkwy

20th Ave

Parsons Blvd

147th St

150th St

149th St

20th Ave

Clintonville St

Francis Lewis Blvd

Willets Point Blvd

678

0   0.2   0.4   0.6 mile
0   0.2   0.4   0.6 kilometer

12 WHITESTONE aND MaLBa: MOVING ON UP

BOUNDARIES: Francis Lewis Park, Clintonville St., Cross Island Pkwy., Boulevard
DISTANCE: 3 miles
SUBWAY: 7 to Main St.–Flushing, transfer to Q15 bus

The Throgs Neck and Whitestone Bridges bracket the neighborhood of Whitestone, located on land jutting into the East River. Dutch colonists sailing into the area supposedly spotted limestone boulders on the shore, hence its name. They paid the Matinecoc tribe one ax for every 50 acres of land per a written agreement of 1684 (whose language and terms were no doubt incomprehensible to the natives). Two defining events happened in the mid-19th century: John D. Locke, the proprietor of a metalware factory, relocated his operation from Brooklyn to Whitestone—where it would employ 300 people at its peak—and the Long Island Rail Road launched service at Whitestone with a station near the village center. The LIRR later added two more stops in Whitestone, one close to the water and another to serve a new development to the west called Malba, making the neighborhood convenient for commuters as well as those out for a day at the beach. All of Whitestone's railroad service was terminated in 1932, and from then on, it developed as a quiet, semi-suburban neighborhood.

● Get off the bus on the Cross Island Pkwy. service road at Clintonville St. Backtrack to the intersection, and take the parkway overpass to proceed north on Clintonville St. The aquamarine onion dome of St. Nicholas Orthodox Church beckons on your right. Continuing north, you have your first glimpse of the Throgs Neck Bridge in the distance to your right. At 14th Rd., on the far corner to your left, the large residence with dormer windows lining its mansard roof was a boardinghouse for employees of John Locke's factory (which was just up Clintonville St.). Across from it, Grace Episcopal was called simply the Whitestone Chapel when it was built in 1858. The neighborhood's oldest church, it was refurbished in 1904 and has a charming interior with a wood-beam ceiling.

● Turn left on 14th Ave. Whitestone has a large Italian American population, so why not satisfy your *appetito* at the Italian deli and *salumeria* on the corner, Corona Park Pork Store?

- Make a right on 150th St., in the midst of Whitestone's small commercial district. Harpell Chemists has been open at this right corner since 1906. Across the street, Freddy's Pizzeria is another local fixture for Italian food. Midblock on your left, the pub at #12-54 has a nicely ornamented exterior courtesy of the defunct First National Bank, which erected the building in 1907. A block farther on your right is the home of the Whitestone Community Ambulance Service, a volunteer agency that's been answering calls 24/7 since 1947. Upon crossing 12th Ave., you have a farmhouse from the 1880s on your left, followed by houses built from 1900 through 1910. Opposite them is a very recent construction: the Holy Cross church, whose parking lot took the place in 2009 of a petite, old-fashioned ex-Methodist church that the Greek Orthodox congregation had used for 35 years. At 11th Ave., the funeral home on your right is a beautiful Victorian dating to 1890.

- Turn left on 11th Ave. Years ago, pilots used the lighted steeple of Immanuel Lutheran Church to guide their planes to the LaGuardia Airport runway; you, instead, have to look up at this charmer, the second-oldest church in Whitestone. Serving the community since 1894, Immanuel Lutheran today proclaims itself "a mosaic ministry": Its website can be read in 15 languages, and its weekly calendar includes Chinese Bible study and Hindi and Tamil worship. This block offers a diversity of its own, lovely older homes interspersed with newer models ranging from unremarkable to rather garish.

- Make a right on 149th St. and again on 10th Ave. The large house on the right corner across 150th St., with its pretty door and oval window, is worth a look. It's one of several homes from the early 1900s on this stretch.

- Walk north on 150th St., even-numbered houses to your left. Across 9th Ave. on your right, the Victorian has a dormer window nestled up to its turret and a large black star on the front facade. Past 8th Ave., the outstanding second house on the left has a lot going on—Tuscan columns and fan-shaped trim on the porch, protruding bay on the second floor, and contrasting shapes of the gables and windows within. Somewhere in this vicinity, Walt Whitman resided from late 1840 into the spring of 1841 while teaching at the Whitestone School. He wrote about Whitestone in correspondence, pleased with his accommodations and proximity to the water but demurring at its residents' "gold-scraping" and "wealth-hunting."

- Make a left on 5th Ave.

- Turn right on 148th St.

- Make a left on 3rd Ave. You're very close to the northernmost point in Queens. Remember, the borough's avenues are numbered from the north. Whitestone is the only place with avenue numbers lower than 5th.

- Just past 147th St. on 3rd Ave., enter Francis Lewis Park, one of the best-sited parks in the city. Follow the path on the right, and as you pass the fourth bench, look beyond it to the house (on 147th St.) with chimney and shutters, said to have been built in the 1760s. Continue down to the water, and go onto the beach if you'd like. In the first few decades of the 20th century, Whitestone flourished as a seaside resort, with yacht clubs, bathing pavilions, and amusements. The graceful Whitestone Bridge (formally, the Bronx-Whitestone Bridge), which has the highest towers of any East River span, opened one day before the 1939 World's Fair. As for the park's namesake, Francis Lewis was the only Queens signer of the Declaration of Independence. The Wales-born Lewis moved to Whitestone after retiring from business in 1765; while residing here, he was elected to the Continental Congress. During the Revolutionary War, the British destroyed Lewis's house and imprisoned his wife, Elizabeth, who died in 1779, probably from ailments incurred in captivity. Ironically, Lewis had made his fortune supplying British troops during the French and Indian War. From the water, go back up on the other side of the park, and exit at its western corner on 3rd Ave., next to the bridge foundations.

- Go to the right on 3rd Ave., walking under the bridge into Malba, a swanky neighborhood (within Whitestone's zip code) developed on land that had been owned by Royal Baking Powder mogul William Ziegler. Malba has no commerce and no public transportation except at its southern reaches around 14th Ave. The real estate partners who created Malba in 1908 arranged the initials of their surnames—Maycock, Avis, Lewis, Bishop, and Alling—into a name for their new community. About 15 houses were constructed in its first decade, including the first one on your left. As you can see across Parsons Blvd. from it, Malba's current inventory of 410 homes includes plenty of recent McMansions.

- Turn right from 3rd Ave. onto Parsons Blvd., which quietly begins its journey south to Jamaica here. (For most of its 6.5 miles, Parsons is a wide commercial thoroughfare.) Eyebrow dormers and a stone chimney punctuate the roof of the second house on your right. The enviable lot on your left as you round the bend features a Mediterranean palazzo, while the houses on the right have a bridge in their backyard. Continue straight down to the water. No yacht-club membership is required to take in the view, from the tops of the Empire State Building and Triborough Bridge to waterfront mansions nearby.

- Go back to the intersection and to the right on Malba Dr., where those waterfront mansions are located. Opposite Summit Pl., note the sailboat on the gate of the arcade linking the house and garage. Three doors farther is a Tudor castle with beautiful stained glass.

- Turn right at the guardhouse, which used to be staffed. Malba homeowners still pay for private security patrol, and they didn't give up ownership of their streets to the city until the 1980s. This road is called Boulevard, and the body of water is Powell's Cove. Malba once had a private beach here. The house at the water's edge with a second-floor patio is one of roughly 100 houses built in Malba in the 1920s. Squawking geese can disturb this spot's serenity. If you hear other bird noise while walking in Malba, look atop utility poles for green monk parrots.

- Make the next left to stay on Boulevard. On your left between North Dr. and Center Dr. stands a 1925 green-roofed villa with multicolored tiling.

- Turn left on Center Dr.

- Turn right on Malba Dr. The MALBA welcome sign on the island at 11th Ave. succeeded a grand fieldstone gate that marked the neighborhood's entry—until it was sacrificed for widening of the Whitestone Expy. in the early 1960s. You will merge onto the highway's service road as Malba Dr. ends one block uphill.

- Turn left on 14th Ave. and cross the overpass. To the right on Parsons Blvd., there's a stop for the Jamaica-bound Q44, which takes you to the 7 in Flushing.

POINTS OF INTEREST

Corona Park Pork Store coronaparkporkstore.com, 150-54 14th Ave., 718-767-2654

Freddy's Pizzeria 12-66 150th St., 718-767-4502

Francis Lewis Park 3rd Ave. and 147th St.

route summary

1. Walk north on Clintonville St. from the Cross Island Pkwy.
2. Turn left on 14th Ave.
3. Turn right on 150th St.
4. Make a left on 11th Ave.
5. Turn right on 149th St.
6. Go right on 10th Ave.
7. Make a left on 150th St.
8. Turn left on 5th Ave.
9. Turn right on 148th St.
10. Make a left on 3rd Ave.
11. Go into Francis Lewis Park.
12. Walk west on 3rd Ave. after leaving the park.
13. Turn right on Parsons Blvd.
14. Follow Malba Dr. south from the river.
15. Make a right onto Boulevard.
16. Turn left on Center Dr.
17. Turn right on Malba Dr., which merges into the Whitestone Expy.
18. Go left on 14th Ave. and right on Parsons Blvd. for the bus.

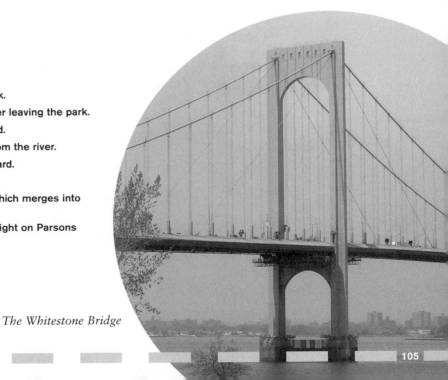

The Whitestone Bridge

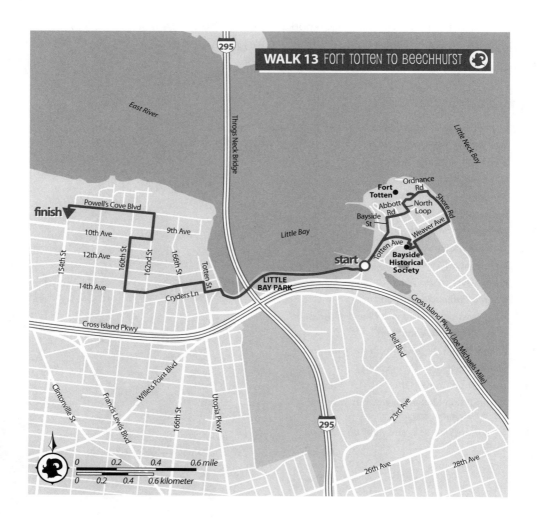

WALK 13 FORT TOTTEN TO BEECHHURST

Throgs Neck Bridge

East River

Little Neck Bay

Ordnance Rd

Fort Totten

Abbott Rd

North Loop

Shore Rd

Bayside St

Weaver Ave

finish

Powell's Cove Blvd

10th Ave

9th Ave

Little Bay

start

Totten Ave

Bayside Historical Society

154th St

12th Ave

160th St

162nd St

166th St

Totten St

14th Ave

Cryders Ln

LITTLE BAY PARK

Cross Island Pkwy (Joe Michaels Mile)

Cross Island Pkwy

Clintonville St

Francis Lewis Blvd

Willets Point Blvd

166th St

Utopia Pkwy

Bell Blvd

23rd Ave

26th Ave

28th Ave

295

0   0.2   0.4   0.6 mile
0   0.2   0.4   0.6 kilometer

13 FORT TOTTEN TO BEECHHURST: GREAT VIEWS ON LITTLE BAY

BOUNDARIES: Fort Totten battery, Shore Rd., Little Bay, 154th St.
DISTANCE: 3.5 miles
SUBWAY: 7 to Flushing–Main St., transfer to Q13 or Q16 bus to Fort Totten

On the north shore of Queens, the land forms small peninsulas between bays of the East River. LaGuardia Airport sits on the westernmost of these peninsulas; Fort Totten is on one farther east, between Little Bay and Little Neck Bay. This decommissioned Army base has been converted into a city park, complete with outdoor swimming pool. The fort was designed in the 1850s, the pre-rifling age, and would never be involved in combat because rifled artillery started to become the norm during the Civil War soon after it was built. (Robert E. Lee had a hand in designing the fort when he was an officer in the Army Corps of Engineers prior to the war.) Its battery wasn't even completed once test shots fired at it proved it could not hold up to rifled attacks. You see the battery and other historic structures while roaming the grounds of Fort Totten. This walk then takes you through a shoreside park en route to Beechhurst, a residential neighborhood that many consider part of Whitestone.

● Both bus routes terminate at the entrance to Fort Totten, close to the Throgs Neck Bridge. Along with the older Fort Schuyler, which is beneath the bridge in the Bronx, Fort Totten was designed to protect New York Harbor from attack via the Long Island Sound. It ended up being used instead by the Army Corps of Engineers for, among other things, weapons development. The silver spheres atop the gate pillars were torpedo mines, manufactured here. Walk straight ahead after entering the fort until you reach the triangle near Bldg. 203. Buried within a grove behind the triangle is Charles Willets, who owned this land before the federal government acquired it. (In present-day Queens geography, Willets Point refers to an area in Flushing near the Mets' ballpark, but that's named for Willets Point Blvd., which runs between there and this original Willets Point.)

- Facing the grave, go right. Bldg. 637 was constructed in the 1890s for an Army Corps of Engineers school (that eventually moved to Washington, DC) and later served as a commissary and then a storehouse. Next to it is the fort's second chapel—the first one from 1870 burned down. Ahead on your right is the former officers' club, a medieval castle just like the one in the Army Corps of Engineers' logo. The Bayside Historical Society, which is headquartered in "the Castle," is dedicated to restoring the 1887 building and archiving Bayside's history. The society always has some photographs and objects on display. You can also go upstairs to the ballroom.

- Upon exiting the Castle, go to your right to see the building next door. It's the only one that was here before the fort—the Willets family's circa-1830 farmhouse, which was moved from its original location nearer the water.

- Head back in the Castle's direction and turn right on Weaver Ave. On your left, the parks department has taken over the former commanding officer's house, which has tall fluted columns and was built opposite the parade grounds (now sports fields) with a balcony from which the commanding officer could watch the parades. Most of the other buildings in this section are used by the city's fire department.

- Turn left at the gazebo at the bottom of the hill. That's Great Neck, in Nassau County, across Little Neck Bay, and your view includes the US Merchant Marine Academy there.

- Fort Totten's battery is at the end of the road, but you have to make a left and enter through the visitors' center. It's in the old ordnance building, behind which you can see doors to the torpedo magazines, where mines like those at the fort entrance were stored. Some torpedo mines were put into the water between Forts Totten and Schuyler during the Spanish-American War but, obviously, never detonated. In addition to awesome views, the battery's intriguing sights include soldiers' graffiti on the tunnel walls, a gunpowder room, a staircase to upper levels that were never built, and iron-shuttered windows from which cannons were to be fired. The battery provided the postapocalyptic setting for Jay Z's video "Run This Town," filmed with Rihanna and Kanye West in 2009.

- Make a right out of the visitors' center. When the road ends, turn left.

- Make a right on Abbott Rd. and a left when it ends, facing the water. Follow the road back to the gate.

- After exiting the fort, walk to the bus stop, then cross the street and enter Little Bay Park. (If this is blocked by construction, continue on the sidewalk away from the fort and turn right at the first traffic light; a path will take you into the park.) Go down to the path next to the water and follow it as it hugs the shoreline, eventually walking beneath the Throgs Neck Bridge, the youngest bridge that spans the East River. Upon its opening in January 1961, Queens' connections to "mainland" New York were complete. It was built to relieve traffic on the Whitestone and Triborough Bridges but, in effect, probably increased traffic—an additional bridge encouraged more people to drive to and from Long Island (even as the toll, originally 25¢, rose to $7.50). As for its name: John Throckmorton owned the neck of land on the Bronx side back in the 1600s, and the name was compressed somewhere along the way. Stay on the path all the way to the park's entrance in Beechhurst.

- Make a left after passing between the pillars, but stay to the right so that you're on Cryders Ln., not Utopia Pkwy. In the 1800s, Mr. Cryder owned much of the land that would be developed after the turn of the century as a residential community named Beechhurst. This is the only road that existed before then. These days Beechhurst is battling "McMansionizing" like so many other Queens neighborhoods; a 2005 rezoning was instituted to reduce instances of replacing older homes with ostentatious contemporary models.

- Turn right on Totten St.

- Make a left on 14th Ave. You're now within Robinwood, which was developed separately from—and later than—Beechhurst, with pricier homes on larger lots. All these distinctions tend to be ignored by outsiders, who would just call the whole area between the bridges Whitestone (it's all the same zip code). But those who live east of 154th St. generally prefer to identify as Beechhurst, and real estate agents keep Robinwood in circulation for the air of exclusivity. The oldest houses are from the 1910s and 1920s, including the side-by-side slate-roofed L-shaped Tudors midblock on your right. Across 166th St., 13th and 14th Aves. converge; stay on 14th, on the left.

- Make a right on 160th St.

- Go right on 10th Ave. As you can see as you approach 162nd St., the northeast corner of Beechhurst contains several high-rise apartment buildings. The largest is directly in front of you. Le Havre was developed by the Levitts of Levittown fame. It was constructed in the 1950s on the last remaining farmland in Beechhurst.

- Turn left on 162nd St. On the far side of 9th Ave., a giant cylinder stands in the parking lot, labeled LE HAVRE; it was the Cryder farm's water tower and had long been out of commission when the apartments were built.

- Make a left on Powell's Cove Blvd., which still has plenty of grand old homes. (In the other direction, at the end of Powell's Cove Blvd. you'd find Wildflower, a red-roofed neo-Tudor mansion built in the 1920s for theatrical producer Arthur Hammerstein after he'd had a big hit with the operetta *Wildflower,* cowritten by his nephew Oscar Hammerstein II, who went on to make musical-theater history with Richard Rodgers. It's been subdivided into condos of the gated community Wildflower Estates.) One reason Hammerstein's house received a landmark designation is that it represents the period when Beechhurst was populated with showbiz folks; other residents in the 1920s included Howard Thurston, Helen Kane, and Harry Richman—all famous in their day but mostly forgotten now. One celebrity for the ages who lived here was Charlie Chaplin, who resided at the Towers apartments on your right at 161st St.

  Continue to 154th St. The shopping center there is the former Whitestone Landing, served by the Long Island Rail Road from 1886 to 1932. If hungry, grab a slice at Cascarino's, a mini-chain of pizzerias within the borough. You can get the Q15 bus back to Flushing on 154th St.

POINTS OF INTEREST

Fort Totten Cross Island Pkwy. and Totten Rd., 718-352-1769

Bayside Historical Society baysidehistorical.org, 208 Totten Ave., 718-352-1548

Little Bay Park Cross Island Pkwy. between Utopia Pkwy. and Totten Rd.

Cascarino's cascarinos.com, 152-59 10th Ave., 718-746-4370

route summary

1. Enter the fort grounds and walk on Totten Ave., bearing right at the triangle.
2. Turn right on Weaver Ave. from the Castle.
3. Make a left on Shore Rd.
4. Turn left on Ordnance Rd. for the battery and visitors center.
5. Turn left on North Loop from Ordnance Rd.
6. Make a right on Abbott Rd.
7. Turn left on Bayside St.
8. Follow Totten Rd. out of the fort, and then enter Little Bay Park on its north side.
9. Walk west on the bayside path.
10. Exit the park at its western end, and head west on Cryders Ln.
11. Make a right on Totten St.
12. Turn left on 14th Ave.
13. Go right on 160th St.
14. Turn right on 10th Ave.
15. Make a left on 162nd St.
16. Go left on Powell's Cove Blvd. to 154th St.

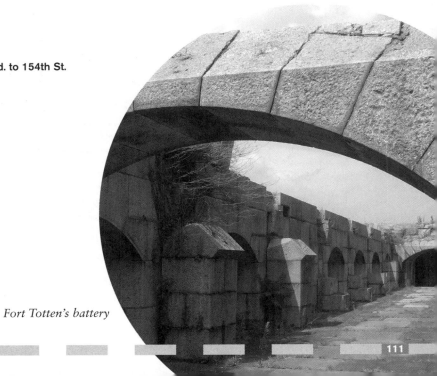

Fort Totten's battery

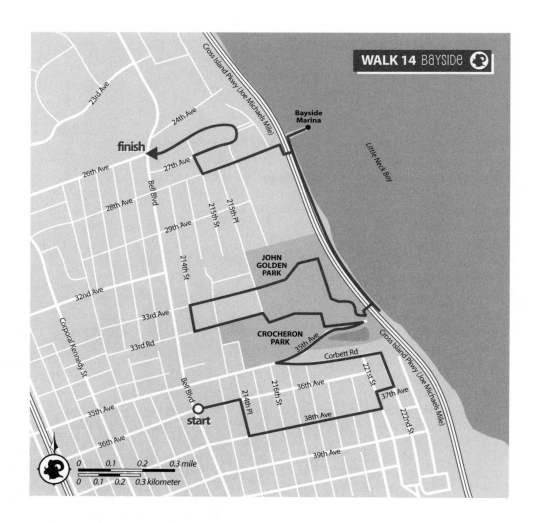

WALK 14 Bayside

Cross Island Pkwy (Joe Michaels Mile)

23rd Ave

24th Ave

Bayside Marina

finish

27th Ave

26th Ave

28th Ave

Bell Blvd

215th Pl

215th St

29th Ave

Little Neck Bay

JOHN GOLDEN PARK

214th St

32nd Ave

33rd Ave

Corporal Kennedy St

33rd Rd

CROCHERON PARK

35th Ave

Corbett Rd

Cross Island Pkwy (Joe Michaels Mile)

221st St

37th Ave

Bell Blvd

start

214th Pl

216th St

36th Ave

38th Ave

222nd St

35th Ave

36th Ave

39th Ave

0   0.1   0.2   0.3 mile
0   0.1   0.2   0.3 kilometer

14 Bayside: so much to admire

BOUNDARIES: 26th Ave., Little Neck Bay, 38th Ave., Bell Blvd.
DISTANCE: 4.2 miles
SUBWAY: 7 to Main St.–Flushing, transfer to Q13 bus to Fort Totten

Bayside contains everything from a glacial pond to a college campus to a suburban-style mall, but it's thought of primarily as a residential neighborhood—and a highly desirable one at that. It encompasses at least half a dozen subdivisions and smaller communities. This walk, for instance, begins in Bellcourt, which was developed from the last parcel of Abraham Bell's farm to be sold off by his descendants. It concludes in exclusive Bayside Gables, to which automobile access is controlled by gate. Throughout Bayside, homes from a century ago stand side by side with McMansions of a much more recent vintage. Its history goes back to colonial times, when it was settled as an eastern offshoot of Flushing. In the 1930s and '40s, a six-lane highway was laid between the neighborhood and its namesake bay. Fortunately, the Cross Island Pkwy. has a few pedestrian overpasses, and one of them ushers you to a wonderful shorefront trail. Between that segment and traipsing through two parks, this route has plenty of off-street walking.

● **Get off the bus on Bell Blvd. at 36th Ave., in front of Redeemer Lutheran Church, established in 1915. A newer arrival, Siloam Reformed Church, worships across 36th Ave. in a building constructed in 1923 for a Masonic lodge. Across Bell Blvd. is a red-roofed mansion made of cobblestones. The 1906 house was landmarked because cobblestone houses are rare and these stones were not cut or shaped in any way. The rear mirrors the front, with three dormer windows above a porch with three wide arches. Now used commercially, the house has not been a single-family residence since the original owner sold it in the early 1920s. On its lawn, a pillar bears the old street names (Bell Ave. and Lamartine Ave.); such gateposts flanked each avenue leading into Bellcourt.**

● **Walk east on 36th Ave. The compact house with a porch on your right dates to the 1930s, though many of its neighbors are much younger. Look up and down the streets, and you'll see that Bayside is full of blocks shared by homes from different eras.**

SCENIC COLLEGE CAMPUSES

Bayside's former Oakland Golf Club was transformed into the campus of **Queensborough Community College,** on 56th Ave. east of Springfield Blvd. Its charming former clubhouse now serves as the QCC Art Gallery, whose exhibitions can run the gamut from Picasso to Chinese pottery to digitally created paintings. The gallery owns an acclaimed African collection. Also open to the public is the Kupferberg Holocaust Resource Center and Archives, which presents exhibits, lectures, and film screenings. In addition, the college is home to the Queensborough Performing Arts Center, a professional touring house for well-known music, comedy, dance, and theater acts, as well as the venue for the annual holiday and spring concerts of the Oratorio Society of Queens, the borough's oldest performing arts group, established in 1927.

Queens College, a four-year school in the City University of New York system, is located at the border of Flushing and Kew Gardens Hills. Its grassy, tree-lined quad is bordered by Spanish Mission–style buildings with Art Deco facade reliefs. At its east end, near the campus entrance at Kissena Blvd. and Melbourne Ave., stands Jefferson Hall, built in 1907 for the delinquent-boys school that occupied the site before the college opened in the 1930s. Opposite Jefferson Hall, look for the boulder outside the Student Union commemorating Walt Whitman's brief tenure teaching at Jamaica Academy, the school located on-site in the early 19th century. At the west end of the quad, Cooperman Plaza features a fountain, a 9/11 memorial garden, and a view of the Manhattan skyline. Art exhibitions are held in the Godwin-Ternbach Museum, and nationally known artists are booked at the college's performing arts center. The Queens Symphony Orchestra, a 60-year-old professional ensemble, performs there regularly.

Sculpture on the grounds of QCC

- Turn right on 214th Pl., which still has 1920s houses.

- Make a left on 38th Ave. and enjoy seven pleasant residential blocks. Since 1896, Sacred Heart of Jesus has built and replaced a series of buildings along this stretch of 38th Ave.—or Warburton Ave., as it was named when the parish was founded.

- Turn left on 221st St., then right on 37th Ave. in front of a quaint 1915 house with scalloped shingles. As you head downhill, you can see what looks like a castle tower ahead on the left. This building has had several uses (it's currently a day-care center) since it was built as a private residence adjacent to a beach. The Cross Island Pkwy. cost Bayside its shorefront; before the highway was constructed in the 1930s, property lines extended right to the water's edge.

- Turn left on 222nd St. Near the end of the block on the right is a property with one brown-shingled house overlooking the shoreline and another brown-shingled house closer to the street. In the 1910s, this was the summer estate of Norma Talmadge, a superstar of the silent-film era, and her husband, Joseph Schenck, also a major figure in the early days of motion pictures (he headed United Artists and 20th Century Fox at their outsets and cofounded the Academy of Motion Picture Arts and Sciences). Talmadge made almost 50 films prior to 1925, had her own production company, and appeared regularly in gossip magazines—but would be in only two talking pictures. (Norma Desmond, the faded movie star in *Sunset Boulevard,* was supposedly named after her.) The Bayside area was an actors' colony before the film industry moved to California. W. C. Fields lived a block away on 223rd St., and other early stars like Theda Bara, Marie Dressler, and May Robson had homes in Bayside.

- Make a left on Corbett Rd., named for the longtime celebrity resident of the second house on your left. Jim Corbett, heavyweight boxing champion of the 1890s, bought this stately Victorian in 1902 as his boxing career was winding down. "Gentleman Jim," who also performed in vaudeville and film, resided here until his death in 1933. The plaque on a boulder near the curb was partly paid for by Madison Square Garden Boxing Inc. Gentleman Jim's house and the home across 221st St. set the stage for this semi-secluded enclave of gracious older residences—with some inauspicious modernizing as well. Bounded by a low stone wall, the corner property across from Corbett's house includes a gazebo, a sculpture of children, and a weathervane-topped cottage.

On your right, past a row of 1980s infill, sits a timber-framed house with praiseworthy landscaping. It faces the westernmost of four consecutive turreted houses. Other fine properties are clustered on this half of the block, including a circa-1920 shingled manse on the right with a pyramidal tower and stone pillars.

● When Corbett Rd. ends near 216th St., loop to your right onto 35th Ave. and enter Crocheron Park. It was created, along with additional acreage, out of the former grounds of a hotel that from 1865 to 1907 (when it burned down) drew both locals and out-of-towners with its resort hospitality and legendary clambakes. Crocherons first settled in the area in the 17th century, and family members have served in the US Congress and State Assembly; Joseph Crocheron, who ran the hotel, was a gambler well known in society circles. His hotel became a Tammany Hall hangout, and Boss Tweed, ringleader of that corrupt political machine, supposedly hid out here after he escaped from jail in 1875.

● Stay on 35th Ave. until you reach Golden Pond, tucked into a corner of the park, on your right. Queens contains quite a few kettle ponds like this, created when chunks of ice deposited by a receding glacier melted.

● From the side of the pond near the ball fields, go up the steps through the woods. At the top, take the path to your left. Make a right after passing the tennis courts, and exit the park in front of the comfort station, on 33rd Rd. at 215th Pl. The fence iron-work alludes to Joseph Crocheron's involvement in horse racing.

● Go straight ahead on 33rd Rd. Opposite the playground at the end of the block is what looks like three adjoining houses with a U-shaped driveway, but they are one house, possibly the oldest in Bayside. It has been traced back to 1852 (although a marker dates it to 1790) and is known as the Cornell-Appleton house—Cornell for early owners of the land, Appleton for the family that bought it in 1905. One of the Appletons who lived here, Charlotte, survived the *Titanic.* Her husband, Edward Dale Appleton, was a grandson of the founder of D. Appleton & Company publishers, which launched *Popular Science* magazine and produced the first US edition of *Alice in Wonderland.*

● Turn right on 214th Pl. or 214th St. (you'll miss some exquisite houses doing the former).

- Turn right on 33rd Ave. It ends at the entrance to John Golden Park. Why are the masks of comedy and tragedy on the plaque? The civic-minded Mr. Golden, namesake of Broadway's Golden Theatre, was a leading theatrical producer and also wrote plays and music. Golden lived in Bayside for 35 years, and the public was welcome to picnic, stroll, and play ball on his estate's grounds even when he was alive.

- Inside the park, walk on the path with the ball fields on your left. Then go right onto the path behind the restroom building into the woodsy area.

- Make a right when the path forks, and you cross into Crocheron Park (there are no signs or gates between the parks). Stay to the left, and past the second gazebo, go down the steps. Take the path on the left (rather than continuing down the stairs) to the pedestrian bridge spanning the highway.

- Cross the bridge, and after you come down the steps, turn around and walk with the water to your right. Joe Michaels Mile, this shore path named for a late local running enthusiast, totals about 2.5 miles between Fort Totten and Northern Blvd., but you'll walk only a little more than a half mile of it.

  Just beyond the next pedestrian bridge is the Bayside Marina, a public facility for boating and recreational fishing. Oystering and clamming were once major businesses on Little Neck Bay but were banned in 1909 due to pollution.

- After visiting the marina, cross the bridge over the highway.

- Walk on 28th Ave. to 215th St. and turn right, entering Bayside Gables, the most posh of Bayside's neighborhoods, with its own security and groundskeeping personnel. Houses date to the 1920s, though some of the original homes have been modernized or replaced with newer models. Sitting on beautifully landscaped lots, they vary in style and feature elements ranging from slate roofs to storybook towers.

- Turn right on 27th Ave. As you pass the grassy traffic island, look below the flagpole for a presidential memorial.

- Go around the bend onto 26th Ave. At Bell Blvd., you see the "gated" entrance to the community.

- Cross Bell Blvd. and wait at a bus stop for the B13 to the Flushing–Main St. 7 station.

POINTS OF INTEREST

Crocheron Park 35th Ave. and 216th St.

John Golden Park 33rd Ave. and 215th Pl.

Joe Michaels Mile Cross Island Pkwy. between Northern Blvd. and Totten Rd.

Bayside Marina baysidemarinany.com, Cross Island Pkwy. and 28th Ave., 718-229-0097

ROUTE SUMMARY

1. Walk east on 36th Ave. from Bell Blvd.
2. Make a right on 214th Pl.
3. Turn left on 38th Ave.
4. Go left on 221st St.
5. Turn right on 37th Ave.
6. Turn left on 222nd St.
7. Turn left on Corbett Rd.
8. Go right on 35th Ave.
9. Walk through Crocheron Park.
10. Take 33rd Rd. from the park.
11. Turn right on 214th St.
12. Make a right on 33rd Ave.
13. Enter John Golden Park, and walk through it and into Crocheron Park.
14. Cross pedestrian bridge over Cross Island Pkwy.
15. Walk north on Joe Michaels Mile.
16. After visiting the marina, cross the highway via the bridge to 28th Ave.
17. Make a right on 215th St.
18. Turn right on 27th Ave.
19. Loop around onto 26th Ave. and proceed to Bell Blvd.

A view from Joe Michaels Mile

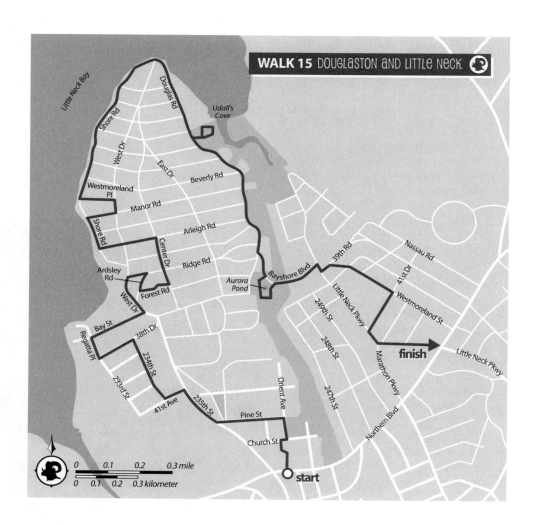

Little Neck Bay

Douglas Rd

Shore Rd

Udall's Cove

West Dr

East Dr

Beverly Rd

Westmoreland Pl

Manor Rd

Shore Rd

Arleigh Rd

Center Dr

Ridge Rd

Ardsley Rd

Aurora Pond

Bayshore Blvd

Forest Rd

West Dr

Bay St

Regatta Pl

38th Dr

234th St

233rd St

41st Ave

235th St

Pine St

Orient Ave

Church St

start

39th Rd

Nassau Rd

41st Dr

Westmoreland St

Little Neck Pkwy

249th St

248th St

247th St

Marathon Pkwy

finish

Little Neck Pkwy

Northern Blvd

0   0.1   0.2   0.3 mile

0   0.1   0.2   0.3 kilometer

15 DOUGLASTON AND LITTLE NECK: SHORE THING

BOUNDARIES: **Douglas Rd., Westmoreland St., Northern Blvd., Shore Rd.**
DISTANCE: **4.3 miles**
SUBWAY: **7 to Main St., transfer to Little Neck–bound Q12 bus**

Before there was Douglas Manor, there was the Douglas manor, a lush 175-acre family estate that New York's social elite visited for yachting, polo, and R&R. In 1906 Rickert-Finlay developers bought the land and created Douglas Manor, the earliest of Queens' 20th-century planned communities. As designed by Rickert-Finlay, Douglas Manor's roads follow the natural curves and slopes of the land, all houses are situated within a mile of the train station, and the waterfront is communally owned and maintained by the homeowners' association. Of Douglas Manor's many spectacular homes, none are more enviably positioned than those on Shore Rd., with their unimpeded views of the boat-filled harbor and Throgs Neck Bridge. Now a landmarked district, Douglas Manor is the focal point of this walk, but it includes other historic and scenic gems of Douglaston and Little Neck, the two neighborhoods on the Little Neck peninsula. At the end, you are but a sixth of a mile from the Nassau County line—and you'll understand why this is known as the gold coast of Queens.

● Get off the bus on Northern Blvd. and 243rd St. Cross Northern and enter the grounds of Zion Church, which has served the community since 1830. This Colonial-style building replaced the original church that burned down in 1924. Wynant Van Zandt III, who retired from Manhattan business and politics to farm on Little Neck Bay, donated the land for it and helped pay to build the first one. Van Zandt died a year after the original building was completed, and he and 10 family members are buried beneath the church's floor. The churchyard is full of prominent early residents of the area.

A couple of graves are of particular note: Facing the front doors, go to the left, and you will see a large cross that says CUTTER. Bloodgood Cutter, the local farmer and mill owner buried here, was a fellow passenger of Mark Twain's on the 1867 voyage to Europe and the Holy Land that Twain chronicled in *The Innocents Abroad.* The eccentric Cutter fancied himself a poet and would frequently share his verses with his not-necessarily-receptive neighbors and acquaintances—a habit Twain mocks in *Innocents Abroad* as "a grievous infliction most kindly meant." Continue around to the other side of the church. When you're next to the chimney, go onto the grass past the Graham grave. Beneath the third large tree on the left, an inscription across two boulders reads, HERE REST THE LAST OF THE MATINECOC. About 30 members of this native tribe, once the largest on Long Island, were reinterred here when their burial ground about a half mile east was absorbed by the widening of Northern Blvd. They'd been buried where they were killed in a 1656 battle against European settlers; earlier skirmishes had made the colonists determined to finish off the Matinecoc, and only a few women, children, and old men survived the slaughter.

● Leave the church property via the nearest exit, on Church St., and walk down Orient Ave.

● Turn left on Pine St., entering the Douglaston Hill historic district, which extends less than two blocks in both directions. The first three houses on your right were all built around 1904 for the same family. The first two were nearly identical originally, but one has since enclosed its front porch; the third is basically a wider version of the other two, with a wraparound porch. The red-shingled house after them was the last of six houses in Douglaston Hill developed speculatively by William and Josephine Hamilton (note the name of the street opposite the house). The Hamiltons' earliest project was #240-45, built in the 1890s and designed by the architect of Zion Church's rectory. Across from it, #240-44 also dates to the 1890s, making these houses the oldest on the street. The Hamiltons lived in the 1900 house at #240-35, a twin of its western neighbor. You head downhill with outstanding circa-1907 homes on your left.

● Cross Prospect Ave. and Douglaston Pkwy. to 235th St., and go to the right. Toward the end of the block, the American Legion hall on your left was constructed in 1906 as a firehouse (complete with signal bell at top) by a volunteer brigade whose duties were eventually superseded by the FDNY. Use the rail-station underpass to get to the other side of the tracks. The Douglas family donated this land to the Long Island Rail Road in 1866 and in return had the station named for them; before then, everywhere on the peninsula was just considered Little Neck.

● Make a left on 41st Ave., then a right on 234th St. On your right, you can see P.S. 98 and the Community Church from the back (they face Douglaston Pkwy.). Then you reach the multitower St. Sarkis church.

● Turn left on 38th Dr.

- Make a right on Regatta Pl., where a beautiful 1870 wood-clad Colonial mansion stands on the left beyond a gated driveway and peeper-deterring tall hedge. The homes on that side have Little Neck Bay as their backyard.

- Turn right on Bay St. Almost all its houses were constructed between 1905 and 1915, and the oldest are the crème de la crème: three consecutive circa-1900 Victorians on your right, starting with the pale yellow house where round and angular towers rise above a wraparound porch. Next door is another Queen Anne with an amalgam of curved and polygonal shapes in its porch, bays, and windows. The house after that offers such picturesque details as horseshoe moldings and windows, decorative shingles, and a conical porch. You saw the rear lawns of this house and the white Colonial with black shutters on 38th Dr. Among the standouts on your left is #205 (it displays this historic address, rather than the current #234-05, on the door), which has white Tudor half-timbering on a pink stucco facade and stained glass windows above an elaborate door pediment.

- Turn left on West Dr., passing two 1920 Colonials on your left—the first with half-moon windows within triangular dormers and the second bearing a copper-covered roof—as you enter Douglas Manor. Its design took cues from the English garden city model, so verdancy and landscaping were important in Douglas Manor, and some of its trees have survived from when the Douglases, who planted many imported varieties, owned the land. At the bend in this road, there's a slate-roofed Tudor cottage on your left; even its garage looks like it came out of a storybook. The next house on that side, at the corner with Alston Pl., is a remnant of when Dutch settlers farmed in the area. The landmarked house, modified and enlarged over the years, was built by Cornelius Van Wyck in 1735 and acquired by Wynant Van Zandt in the early 1800s. From West Dr., you're looking at the back of the house, as it faces the bay.

- Go right onto Ridge Rd. opposite the Van Wyck house. At Ardsley Rd., thanks to the corner lot's elevation, you get a good look at the wood-shingled house that's busy with dormers and windows. If you think this blue trim is bright . . .

- Turn right onto Ardsley Rd. and get a load of the cotton-candy color next door. Positioned diagonally to the corner with Forest Rd., the house has wings that could stand alone as cottages. This pink confection contrasts sharply with the plain, boxy dwelling across Forest Rd. That 1919 home with a multi-dormered mansard roof is said to have been designed by McKim, Mead & White, preeminent architects of New York City's Gilded Age.

- Make a left on Forest Rd. Across Cedar Ln., you are looking at the rear of a white mansion with a Doric-columned porch. Continue up to Center Dr., and you'll see that the front is virtually identical. Such symmetry is the hallmark of Greek Revival homes, though the bracketed attic windows, second-story window lintels, and cupola, among other things, represent an Italianate influence. Constructed in the late 1840s, it's known as the Allen-Beville House for Benjamin P. Allen, who had it built on what was then a 16-acre estate, and television executive Hugh M. Beville, who owned it when it was landmarked. (Allen is buried in Zion's churchyard.)

- Turn left on Center Dr., facing a house with a lunette window. One block farther on your left is another gracious white house with a distinctive window, this one Palladian-style above a semicircular portico.

- Make a left on Arleigh Rd. Downhill, close to the water, you find some of the earliest houses built for the Douglas Manor development: The last two houses on your left and the house on your right at Shore Rd. all date from 1908 to 1910.

- Turn right onto Shore Rd. On the far side of Hollywood Ave., #202 looks more modern than its 1919 construction date, thanks to alterations. Expressionist artist George Grosz lived here for 20 years after fleeing when the Nazis came to power in his native Germany, and for a while theater director Erwin Piscator, another German expat, stayed with him. After Grosz moved out (to return to Germany) in the late 1950s, the home was purchased by Chilean pianist Claudio Arrau. Both Arrau and Grosz gave lessons inside this house. Grosz's drawings and paintings of Douglaston have sold at auctions.

- Make a right on Manor Rd. Atop the rise at West Dr., the Douglaston Club occupies a Greek Revival mansion that passed through the hands of several major Douglaston figures. The house was built in 1819 for Wynant Van Zandt, purchased in 1862 by George Douglas, and eventually owned by his son William. The property later served as the Douglaston Inn. The Douglases were yachtsmen, and their boat Sappho won the inaugural America's Cup in 1871. The first Douglaston yacht club was organized in the 1880s with a "floating" clubhouse that would be towed into the middle of the bay and anchored. That group didn't last (neither did its clubhouse, which blew away in a nor'easter), and its successor is based at the Douglaston Club, which also features tennis courts, a swimming pool, bowling alley, and dining room. John McEnroe, who grew up a block away on Manor Rd., started playing tennis here at the Douglaston Club.

- Turn left on West Dr. and left on Westmoreland Pl., heading back toward the waterfront.

- Make a right on Shore Rd. The second house's wings were angled to optimize views. This 1916 mansion was named Coo-ee (a sound made in the Australian bush to call for attention) by its Australian-born original owner, Annette Kellerman, who had a multifaceted and precedent-setting career. After winning swim races in her teens, Kellerman made the first attempts by a woman to swim the English Channel. She subsequently became a star of the early movies (filmed at the Astoria studios), usually playing a mermaid, and performed in water shows on stage. She is credited with popularizing both synchronized swimming and one-piece swimsuits for women, and she was arrested for indecency for wearing a one-piece rather than the traditional dress with pantaloons.

- A half block farther, you come to the Douglas Manor dock and beach, open only to residents. Past Warwick Ave., the second house evokes its 1913 Arts and Crafts roots in its ell layout, wavy slate roof, and unusually shaped stucco chimney. Other singular features of the homes on this road include a darling conservatory behind the house on the far corner of Knollwood Ave. and, on the next block, a white house with semicircular trellises between its first- and second-floor windows.

202 Shore Rd.

- Cross Bayview Ave., where #1102 employs a pebble surface. Its roof of cedar shingles processed to resemble thatch was most likely copied from two houses away, #1114, built in 1907 in the style of an English cottage.

- As you come around the bend, Shore Rd. turns into Douglas Rd. After passing the Douglas Manor Association's (DMA) private park between Kenmore and Richmond Rds., watch on the left for the UDALL'S WILDLIFE PRESERVE sign. Take this short nature detour, going to the left on the path inside the woods and then making a right when you're facing the DMA park. Follow the path until it forks and go to the right, then down to your left to reach the cove. If it feels like the ends of the earth, well, it is—at least as far as New York City is concerned: This is the easternmost point in the city. Named for a local 19th-century mill owner, Udall's Cove only came under the parks department's purview in the 1970s, in response to a citizen conservation effort. The preserve now comprises a corridor of 40-plus acres between here and Northern Blvd., some of it inaccessible or located behind private homes, with about a half dozen entry points. Here at the head of the cove, a tidal salt marsh thrives around the narrow inlet between Douglaston and Great Neck in Nassau County. The red-roofed Douglas Rd. house overlooking the marsh was the home of Aurora Gareiss, who launched the conservation campaign. Go left as you leave the cove. After stepping over some concrete relics, make a left any time the path divides, and it will lead you back to Douglas Rd.

- Proceed south on Douglas Rd. On the next block, the gray New England–style cottage was designed in 1916 by Josephine Wright Chapman, one of the few women to make a living in architecture at the time. Chapman came to New York from Boston, where she'd designed a few churches and a Harvard dorm but was still rejected for membership in the American Institute of Architects. Douglas Manor has the largest collection of her homes—eight in all, including the next two on the right heading up Grosvenor St. This corner home's property includes the fenced-in lawn across Douglas Rd. Continue walking on Douglas.

- After Ridge Rd., go to the left down Bayshore Blvd. at the UDALL'S COVE PARK sign. Just past the first buildings, Aurora Pond will be on your right. This is another feature of Udall's Park, a freshwater wetland named for Aurora Gareiss. A creek that flows to the cove (underground part of the way) was dammed in this area when the road you're on was paved, thus creating the pond. I recommend the nature trail that starts on either side of it. When you're finished walking around the pond, continue in the direction you'd been going on Bayshore Blvd., or 39th Ave., as it's known on the Little Neck side (some locals just call it "the back road").

- At the top of the hill is Little Neck's train station. Make a right on Little Neck Pkwy. and cross the tracks.

- Go left on 39th Rd., followed promptly by a right onto Westmoreland St.—the central road of Westmoreland, which Rickert-Finlay developed around the same time it created Douglas Manor. Among the first houses were those on the far left corners of 40th and 41st Aves.

- Make a right on 41st Dr.

- Turn left onto Little Neck Pkwy., coming around P.S. 94. A monument in front of the school pays tribute to those from the area who served in World War I. Soon after the war ended, Little Neck and Douglaston held their first Memorial Day parade, and it's still a major annual event for the community. Organizers say it's the largest Memorial Day parade in the country, and the governor and mayor often attend it.

- Stay on Little Neck Pkwy. to Northern Blvd., where you have a view of the Art Moderne bank with an eagle and clock embedded in its facade, and beyond it, the two steeples of the Community Church of Little Neck. Get the Flushing-bound Q12 bus on the north side of the boulevard.

POINTS OF INTEREST

Udall's Wildlife Preserve Douglas Rd. and Richmond Rd.

Aurora Pond Udall's Cove Park, Bayshore Blvd. and Douglas Rd.

rouTe summary

1. Walk through the Zion churchyard to Orient Ave.
2. Make a left on Pine St.
3. Turn right on 235th St.
4. Cross the LIRR tracks to 41st Ave., and head west.
5. Make a right on 234th St.
6. Turn left on 38th Dr.
7. Turn right on Regatta Pl.
8. Make a right on Bay St.
9. Turn left on West Dr.
10. Turn right on Ridge Rd.
11. Go right on Ardsley Rd.
12. Make a left on Forest Rd.
13. Go left on Center Dr.
14. Turn left on Arleigh Rd.
15. Make a right on Shore Rd.
16. Make a right on Manor Rd., a left on West Dr., and a left on Westmoreland Pl.
17. Turn right on Shore Rd., which becomes Douglas Rd.
18. Fork left onto Bayshore Blvd.
19. Make a right on Little Neck Pkwy., a left on 39th Rd., and a right on Westmoreland St.
20. Turn right on 41st Dr.
21. Go left on Little Neck Pkwy. and continue to Northern Blvd.

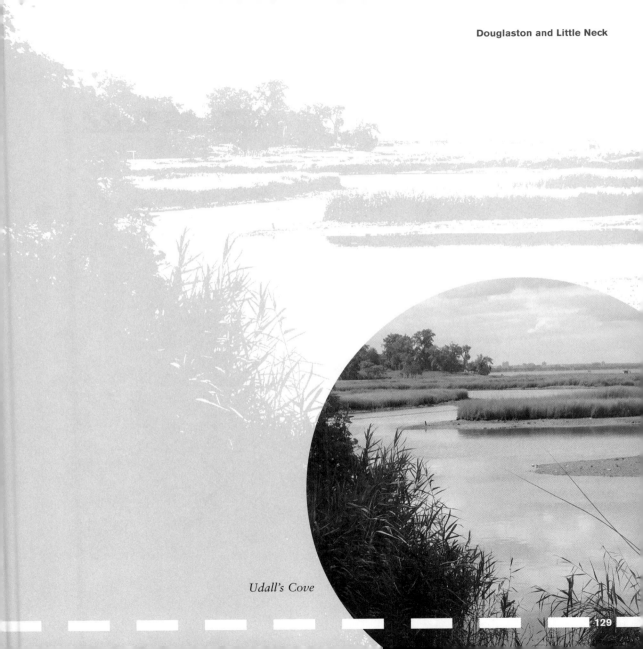

Udall's Cove

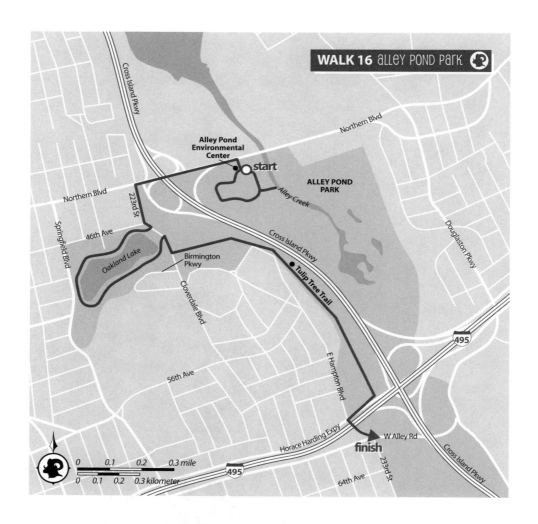

WALK 16 ALLEY POND PARK

Alley Pond Environmental Center

start

ALLEY POND PARK

Alley Creek

Northern Blvd

Cross Island Pkwy

223rd St

Northern Blvd

Springfield Blvd

46th Ave

Oakland Lake

Birmington Pkwy

Cloverdale Blvd

Cross Island Pkwy

Tulip Tree Trail

Douglaston Pkwy

495

56th Ave

E Hampton Blvd

W Alley Rd

finish

233rd St

Cross Island Pkwy

Horace Harding Expy

495

64th Ave

0   0.1   0.2   0.3 mile
0   0.1   0.2   0.3 kilometer

16 alley pond park: ecological wonderland

BOUNDARIES: Northern Blvd., Alley Creek, W. Alley Rd., Oakland Lake
DISTANCE: 3 miles
SUBWAY: 7 to Main St.–Flushing, transfer to Q12 bus to Little Neck

Alley Pond Park, the second-largest park in Queens, is an unusual specimen. First of all, there's its shape: 655 noncontiguous acres approximating an alley—with a couple of nooks off to one side—that extends about 2 miles south from Little Neck Bay. Highways and local roads slice through it, and parts of it are in Bayside, others in Douglaston. Despite all this, Alley Pond Park is an ecological wonderland, with salt marshes, glacial ponds, and forests within its borders. And it's an outstanding specimen of Queens' geologic history. Hills and boulders in the park are a product of the terminal moraine, the accumulation of rock and sand left behind by receding glaciers 20,000 or so years ago. Chunks of glacial ice made depressions in the land that today are ponds. Alley Pond Park is also a specimen of conservation. Much has been done over the last few decades to rehabilitate land suffering due to neglect or development and to protect natural habitats that were being destroyed. Alley Pond Environmental Center (APEC), where this walk begins, has been a linchpin of the conservation efforts since the 1970s.

● APEC is on a stretch of Northern Blvd. with no cross streets, homes, or businesses, so if you're not sure exactly when to signal for the bus to stop, let the driver know where you want to disembark (it's shortly after the Cross Island Pkwy.). There's a stop in front of the center.

Walk behind the APEC building and get on the wooden boardwalk to your left. As you come around the bend, a salt marsh opens up on your left. Alley Creek runs through it, all the way to Little Neck Bay on the other side of Northern Blvd. This is a tidal creek, meaning that the water level fluctuates (by as much as 6 feet, for this particular creek) with the moon's gravitational pull. It is also brackish, containing both freshwater and saltwater. On your right, diminutive Cattail Pond is fed by a spring. There are times when the water is completely covered by cattails and duckweed, and it takes a muskrat swimming through to clear the surface.

- Follow the boardwalk to the left to reach the viewing platform over the creek. The word *alley* was first attached to this area as the nickname of the route colonial Long Islanders would take to and from Brooklyn (where they could get Manhattan-bound ferries).

- After leaving the deck, step off the boardwalk and onto the meadow trail to your left. Proceed onto the wooden planks, which lead you to a grove with a red oak tree (it's labeled) on your right. Alley Pond Park encompasses natural woodlands, but this is what's known as a forest fragment: Its growth has thinned out as trees died because of motor vehicle pollution, among other factors.

- Take the wood-plank path to the right, which goes around Windmill Pond, coated seasonally with algae and wreathed with flora ranging from berry vines to maple trees to a weeping willow.

- Stay on the path alongside the pond, then watch on your right for the windmill. Locals like to think of this as a 19th-century windmill because a grassroots organization worked hard in the 1980s to salvage a 110-year-old Douglaston windmill by getting it moved to this site—only to see it destroyed by arson not long after. This replica now pumps groundwater that the park uses.

WHAT ELSE ALLEY POND PARK OFFERS

The places covered in this walk are all within the park's north section. Playgrounds, ball fields, and tennis courts are in the southern half. Also in the park south of 67th Ave., you can follow marked nature trails through woods and around small ponds. In addition, Alley Pond has a recreational facility that no other NYC park does: a ropes course. The **Alley Pond Adventure Course,** which opened in 2007, includes a zip line, balance platform, climbing wall, pole walk, cables for hanging from or walking on, and various other challenges. It is open to the public on Sundays May–November (reservations required July–August) and is available by reservation at other times for school and corporate groups. The park entrance at Cloverdale Blvd. on 73rd or 76th Ave. is the closest one to the course. For golfers both regular and "mini," the Alley Pond Golf Center (located just east of the environmental center, at 232-01 Northern Blvd.) features a driving range and putt-putt course.

- Follow the path to the left behind the windmill to a log cabin, where classes and special events are held. From there, walk past the picnic tables and parking lot to the entrance of the APEC building. The center displays old area photos and nature-related artwork and, most irresistibly, houses a menagerie. Go inside to visit a hedgehog, a chinchilla, ferrets, rabbits, snakes, lizards, parakeets, and other critters.

- Upon exiting APEC, make a left on Northern Blvd. and walk the equivalent of about three blocks, carefully crossing highway exit/entry ramps.

- Turn left on 223rd St., then left on Cloverdale Blvd. To your right is the terrace overlooking Oakland Lake, the largest of Alley Pond Park's glacial ponds. Queens is full of such kettle ponds, as they're known geologically, and many have needed remediation. Oakland Lake's problem began when the waterways feeding it were filled in with cement. Later the lake was essentially drained under a mosquito-control project, and plant life on its shores was disrupted by construction of buildings and roadways nearby. But now you will see the stunning result of its revitalization.

- Proceed counterclockwise around the pond. The name Oakland comes from the Oaks, a vast estate-turned-nursery formerly in the area. The lake had other names in the past and had other uses too, including colonial-era millpond and water source for the old village of Flushing. Today, it is a protected wetlands and state-designated significant habitat.

- Stay on the path all the way around the lake, perhaps playing hide-and-seek with the resident swan en route. When you've returned to your starting point, make a right on Cloverdale Blvd.

- Before you reach a cross street, go into the woods on your left marked by an ALLEY POND PARK sign. This Tulip Tree Trail, like Oakland Lake, immerses you in nature despite car traffic close by. Approximately half of the park's acreage is forest, with mostly oak, maple, and beech varieties, but this section is dominated by tulip trees— no relation to the flower; they're in the magnolia family. Most notably, these woods contain what is believed to be NYC's oldest and tallest living organism: a tree called the Alley Pond Giant that's estimated to be at least 350 years old and possibly as old as 450. It was nearly 134 feet at last measurement—taller than the Statue of Liberty head to toe.

- The trail ends at E. Hampton Blvd. To conclude with a piece of Alley Pond Park's human history, turn left and cross over the Long Island Expy. When E. Hampton Blvd. becomes W. Alley Rd. at 233rd St., cross to the other side and look down for a boulder with a plaque, commemorating George Washington's 1790 journey to Long Island to thank the people who'd aided the war effort.

- Cross back on W. Alley Rd. and wait at the bus stop on that side for the Jamaica-bound Q30, which connects with the F, E, J, and Z trains.

POINTS OF INTEREST

Alley Pond Environmental Center alleypond.com, 228-06 Northern Blvd., 718-229-4000
Alley Pond Park (Oakland Lake and Tulip Tree Trail) Cloverdale Blvd. and 46th Ave.

ROUTE SUMMARY

1. From APEC on Northern Blvd., follow trails and go into the center.
2. Walk west on Northern Blvd. from APEC.
3. Turn left on 223rd St.
4. Turn left on Cloverdale Blvd. and walk around Oakland Lake.
5. Go south on Cloverdale Blvd.
6. Make a left onto Alley Pond Park's Tulip Tree Trail.
7. Turn left on E. Hampton Blvd. where the trail ends.
8. Proceed to intersection of W. Alley Rd. and 233rd St. to view plaque and then get the bus.

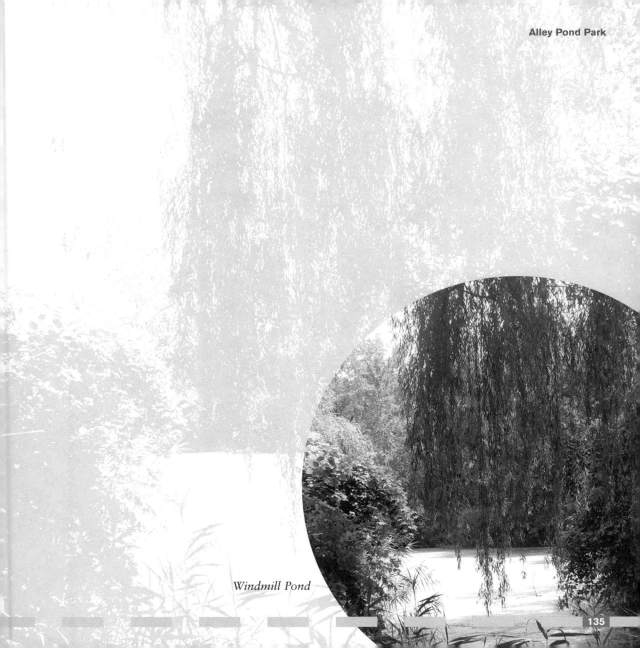

Windmill Pond

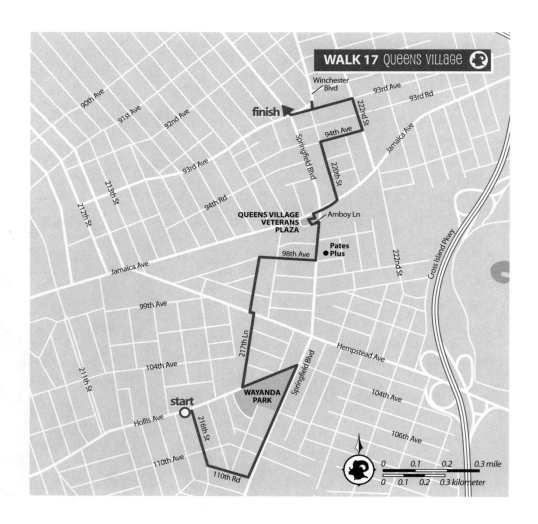

Winchester Blvd

finish

93rd Ave

93rd Rd

222nd St

94th Ave

220th St

Jamaica Ave

Springfield Blvd

93rd Ave

94th Rd

213th St

212th St

94th Rd

QUEENS VILLAGE
VETERANS
PLAZA

Amboy Ln

Pates
Plus

98th Ave

222nd St

Cross Island Pkwy

Jamaica Ave

99th Ave

217th Ln

104th Ave

211th St

Hempstead Ave

104th Ave

WAYANDA
PARK

Springfield Blvd

106th Ave

start

216th St

Hollis Ave

110th Ave

110th Rd

90th Ave

91st Ave

92nd Ave

0   0.1   0.2   0.3 mile

0   0.1   0.2   0.3 kilometer

17 Queens Village: Familiar Name, Unfamiliar Territory

BOUNDARIES: 93rd Ave., 222nd St., 110th Rd., 216th St.
DISTANCE: 2.2 miles
SUBWAY: F to 179th St., transfer to Queens Village–bound Q2 bus

You don't get much farther off the beaten tourist path than Queens Village. It's out in the eastern reaches of the borough, surrounded by residential neighborhoods that don't receive many outside visitors. And what's with that redundant name, anyway? The neighborhood was Queens—yeah, just Queens—until the Long Island Rail Road insisted on clarity and tacked "Village" onto the name of the station in 1924. The LIRR gets to Manhattan in just half an hour, so Queens Village is really not as remote as it may seem. Nonetheless, this is a semiadventurous walk in that it's not a place tailor-made for sightseeing. It has some quirky history: The National Pigeon Shooters Association built a park in the area, complete with grandstand and pavilion, in 1899. The Grand American, an annual shooting competition held there, was a big deal—for three years. Then people started to lose interest in live target shooting, and the whole enterprise went bankrupt in 1902. A community called Bellaire, developed on the old shooting grounds, constitutes the western half of Queens Village. This walk stays in Queens Village proper, east of 212th St.

- Before reaching Queens Village, you get a tour of another neighborhood, Hollis, while the bus rides along Hollis Ave. Get off on Hollis Ave. at 216th St.

- Make a right on 216th St. Walk one long and one short block of tidy, quiet residences—enough variety and vintage for a pleasant stroll. Most of Queens Village is zoned for single- and two-family homes and still has a decent stock from the 1920s and 1930s.

- Go left onto 110th Rd., all identical models on your right after the first house.

- Cross Springfield Blvd. to the Little Sisters of the Poor gate. The stone wall limits your view, but the property is worth a peek as a longstanding, not to mention bucolic, member of the community. The Little Sisters, an order founded in Brittany, France,

QUEENS COUNTY FARM MUSEUM

Queens still has a farm—a real working farm, 47 acres that have been continuously cultivated since 1697. Not surprisingly, it's the only farm left in New York City from colonial times. And rather than shrinking, it has expanded, in terms of both what's grown there and what's accessible to the public. The Queens County Farm Museum, on Little Neck Pkwy. just north of Union Tpke., is open every day, and admission is free. (It's just one neighborhood, and about 2 miles, from Queens Village; to visit after the walk, take a northbound Q27 on Springfield Blvd., and transfer to the Q46 at Union Tpke.)

Very informative tours are given in the 18th-century farmhouse. The property also encompasses an herb garden, fruit orchard, livestock pastures, functional windmill, chicken coop, beehives, flower beds, a vineyard, and fields where dozens of types of vegetables are grown organically. Cows, sheep, pigs, and goats live at the farm. Hayrides are offered on weekends spring–fall. A children's garden invites you to touch, smell, and taste the plantings. The farm's produce is sold on-site June–October, and its eggs, wine, honey, and wool yarn are sold year-round in the gift shop. Special events held annually at the farm include open-hearth dinners, a Native American powwow, an antique-car show, and the Queens County Fair. In the fall, there's a corn maze, pumpkin patch, and Halloween haunted house. And volunteers are always welcome to help with farming. Besides being a unique attraction for NYC, the Queens County Farm Museum offers a unique sight: Where else do you see cows grazing and corn growing with high-rise buildings as their backdrop?

opened this convent in 1902. Novices live here for two years before going to work at a Little Sisters home for low-income seniors. One such home is located on this property.

- Facing the Little Sisters, go to your left on Springfield Blvd. Once past 107th Ave., follow the Flemish gables of P.S. 34 on your left. The illustrious 1905 structure, dramatically sited on a triangular lot with an expansive front lawn, sports five front gables with scrolls and spheres. The monument in front of the school pays tribute to those from the area who served in World War I, its egalitarian inscription mentioning both "the sons and daughters."

- Turn left onto Hollis Ave., with the school to your left. Behind the school, Wayanda Park is one of Queens' oldest, as it opened in 1912, a year after Queens got its own parks commissioner. The park was developed on a potter's field, and perhaps contritely was given the name Wayanda, reportedly from an American Indian term for "place of happy hearts." Across the avenue, Saints Joachim & Anne is the parish that brought the Little Sisters of the Poor to Queens Village. German and Irish immigrants founded the church in the late 1890s, but it has offered Mass in Creole since the 1970s and is now a hub for the borough's Haitian community.

- Make a right on 217th Ln. One block north of Hempstead Ave., St. Joseph's Episcopal Church recalls the village's rural flavor when the congregation was established in 1870, though this cute shingled chapel was built in the 20th century. The ogee arches of the parish house's porch (next door) echo the church doorway. On the next block, the Victorian on the right is one of the neighborhood's older houses.

- Turn right on 98th Ave., mostly industrial here close to the parallel train tracks. At the corner of 218th St., the Elks lodge, with its seemingly decapitated tower, used to be the Queens Lyceum, home to the local garden club and a semiprofessional theater.

- Turn left on Springfield Blvd. At Pates Plus bakery, on your right, you can try the flaky-crust meat patty (*pate*) that's a Haitian staple.

- After passing beneath the train tracks, make a left on Amboy Ln. Note that in addition to QUEENS VILLAGE, the station is labeled LITTLE PLAINS, the neighborhood's name in the colonial era. Go to your right into Veterans Plaza park. The granite monument was

erected in memory of World War II soldiers from Queens Village and adjacent Belle-
rose, and a block was added later to honor Vietnam and Korea losses. Turn and walk
toward the pergola and flagpole, then exit the park to your left onto Jamaica Ave.

● **Make a right on Jamaica Ave.** Across the intersection at Springfield Blvd. stands
Queens Reformed Church, affectionately called the Old White Church. How old? It's
been here since 1858—when the area was still known as Brushville, after Thomas
Brush, a blacksmith who opened a number of businesses. Opposite the church, the
mammoth pilastered facade of All Nations Apostolic Temple reveals its past as the
Queens Theatre, which opened in 1927, seating 2,500 for movie and vaudeville acts.

● **Turn left on 220th St.**

● **Make a right on 94th Ave.**

● **Turn left on 222nd St.** Inside the house on the right corner before you cross 93rd Rd.,
Albert Snyder was killed in March 1927 by his wife, Ruth, and her married lover,
Judd Gray—a murder that inspired *Double Indemnity, The Postman Always Rings
Twice, Body Heat,* and pretty much every other story where a femme fatale lures
a smitten sap into offing her husband. Ruth had indeed taken out an insurance policy
on her husband with a double-indemnity clause (twice the payout in the case of
death by nonnatural causes). In police questioning and at their trial, Ruth and Gray
each asserted the other was the instigator. They were both convicted and sentenced
to the electric chair. A photograph of Ruth at the moment of her execution, which
ran on the front page of the *Daily News,* caused as much buzz as the killing.

● **Turn left on 93rd Ave.**

● **At 220th St.** use the crosswalk to reach the white chapel of Our Lady of Lourdes,
which was modeled on country churches that the parish's founding minister saw in
France while serving as Army chaplain during World War I. Its non-English worship,
including a weekly Spanish service and occasional Masses in Tagalog, Creole, Por-
tuguese, and Tamil, is held here. Go past the front door to the Winchester Blvd. side,
where there's a grotto, as you may expect for a church with Lourdes in its name.

140

● **Return to 220th St. and proceed on 93rd Ave. to the next intersection. Turn right onto Springfield Blvd. In front of Our Lady of Lourdes's newer church (where Mass is in English), take the Q1 bus to the F train at 179th St.**

POINTS OF INTEREST

Wayanda Park Hollis Ave. and Robard Ln.

Pates Plus patesplus.com, 97-15 Springfield Blvd., 718-468-9868

Queens Village Veterans Plaza Jamaica Ave. and Springfield Blvd.

ROUTE SUMMARY

1. Walk south on 216th St. from Hollis Ave.
2. Go left on 110th Rd.
3. Head north on Springfield Blvd.
4. Make a left on Hollis Ave.
5. Turn right on 217th Ln.
6. Turn right on 98th Ave.
7. Turn left on Springfield Blvd.
8. Make a left on Amboy Ln.
9. Walk through Veterans Plaza.
10. Turn right on Jamaica Ave.
11. Make a left on 220th St.
12. Turn right on 94th Ave.
13. Turn left on 222nd St.
14. Go left on 93rd Ave.
15. Cross avenue at 220th St., go around to Winchester Blvd., and then resume walking west on 93rd Ave.
16. Make a right on Springfield Blvd.

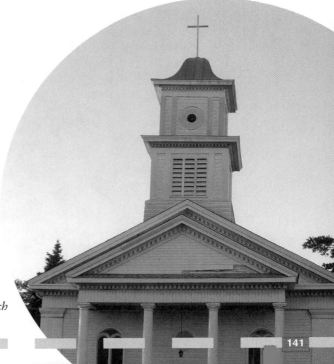

Queens Reformed Church

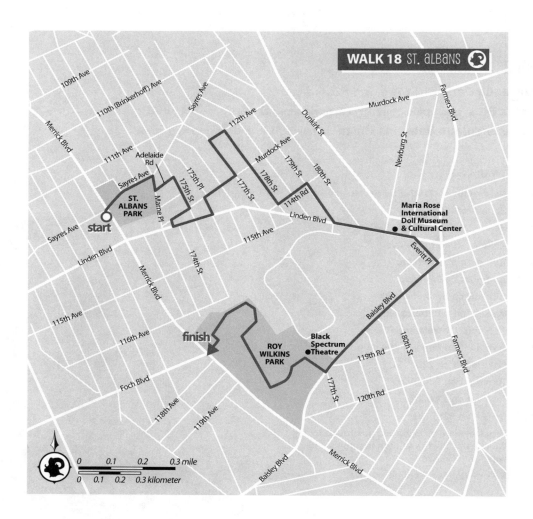

109th Ave

110th (Brinkerhoff) Ave

Sayres Ave

112th Ave

Dunkirk St

Murdock Ave

Farmers Blvd

Merrick Blvd

111th Ave

Adelaide Rd

Sayres Ave

175th Pl

175th St

Marne Pl

177th St

178th St

Murdock Ave

179th St

180th St

Newburg St

ST. ALBANS PARK

start

114th Rd

Linden Blvd

Maria Rose International Doll Museum & Cultural Center

Sayres Ave

Linden Blvd

115th Ave

115th Ave

174th St

Merrick Blvd

Everitt Pl

Baisley Blvd

116th Ave

finish

ROY WILKINS PARK

Black Spectrum Theatre

119th Rd

180th St

Farmers Blvd

Foch Blvd

177th St

120th Rd

118th Ave

119th Ave

Baisley Blvd

Merrick Blvd

0   0.1   0.2   0.3 mile

0   0.1   0.2   0.3 kilometer

18 ST. ALBANS: ALL THAT JAZZ

BOUNDARIES: 112th Ave., Everitt Pl., Baisley Blvd., Merrick Blvd.
DISTANCE: 2.8 miles
SUBWAY: E, J, Z to Jamaica Center–Parsons/Archer, transfer to Q4, Q5, Q84, or Q85 bus

"They all lived here." So says an outdoor mural that you see along this walk. Who were "they"? Black celebrities, primarily jazz entertainers. Beginning in the 1940s, St. Albans was home to such superstars of jazz as John Coltrane, Ella Fitzgerald, and Count Basie, along with other successful but less famous musicians. This wasn't a fleeting phenomenon, either: Illinois Jacquet, master of the "screeching" tenor sax, and bassist Milt "The Judge" Hinton were St. Albans residents of five decades when they passed away in 2004 and 2000, respectively. Jazz musicians even played a part in integrating the neighborhood, specifically its upscale community Addisleigh Park: When racial covenants barring Addisleigh Park home sales to nonwhites were challenged (and upheld) in state court in the 1940s, several black families—including Count Basie's—were already living there. Such covenants would be abolished with the US Supreme Court's 1948 *Shelley v. Kraemer* decision, and Addisleigh Park has now been landmarked by the city for its African American heritage as well as its architectural beauty.

- Take any of the buses at the start of their route on Archer Ave. in Jamaica. As the bus goes south on Merrick Blvd., watch after passing 110th Ave. for the unique steeple of the Greater Allen African Methodist Episcopal Cathedral, a colossal concrete obelisk-and-cone hybrid adjoining the $23 million church complex. Get off the bus at Sayres Ave., where the congregation's former home has been converted to its Shekinah Youth Chapel. The Greater Allen AME megachurch claims to be Queens' second-largest employer (after Kennedy Airport), as it runs an assisted-living facility, affordable housing, a school, and other enterprises. Its longtime pastor Floyd Flake served in the US Congress.

- Cross Merrick Blvd. and walk east on Sayres Ave. next to St. Albans Park. The A-frame building you see across the park is St. Albans Congregational Church. That shape is repeated on your left, in the gables and entry vestibules of the circa-1930 row houses. Some of the houses have stained glass windows on the first floor or a triangular oriel window on the second. A copper cupola tops each corner unit, and #173-19 at the end of the two blocks bears a plaque identifying its famous former resident. Fats Waller was one of the first celebrities, and the first black person, to move to Addisleigh Park; the major influx of jazz artists didn't occur until after his untimely death from pneumonia in 1943.

● Make a right on Marne Pl. and a left on Adelaide Rd. The last house on the left was the home for more than 40 years of Count Basie, the bandleader, composer, and pianist. He and his wife, Catherine, attended the Congregational Church and invited kids in the neighborhood to use their swimming pool.

● Go right on 175th St. The house at the far corner of 113th Ave. has many storybook elements in its entryway alone. Plus, it used to be the residence of Mercer Ellington, a trumpeter who played in and managed the Duke Ellington Orchestra, and then led it after his father Duke's death. At the end of the block on the left, brick, half-timbering, stucco, and slate come together in a striking asymmetrical composition that involves a gable-within-a-gable-within-a-gable.

● Turn right on Murdock Ave. Go to the left at 174th St., walking around the ADDISLEIGH PARK sign, and make a left on Linden Blvd. On the great corner property at 175th St., in between its enclosed porch and cone-shaped portal, delicate arched windows flank a prominent chimney. From Linden Blvd., you can see a tri-dormered Colonial on 175th St. with tall Corinthian columns forming a semicircular portico. Stories have circulated that this was Babe Ruth's summer home after he retired, but no records (or anybody's memories) substantiate them. The rumors probably grew out of Ruth's connection to St. Albans: He was a regular at the golf course that used to be off Linden in the other direction. As you continue along the boulevard, the next corner property on your left has a wonderful round tower faced in cut stone that contains only stairs. The house has had two well-known residents. James Brown, the R&B and civil-rights icon, lived here in the 1960s; before then, it was the residence of Cootie Williams, a jazz trumpeter who cowrote "'Round Midnight" with Thelonious Monk.

● Turn left on 175th Pl., noting the wrought iron driveway gates of the former James Brown house. The only other property on this side of the block is the corner Murdock Ave. home where boxing champion Joe Louis got married on Christmas Day 1955. On your right, adjacent houses offer up cute quarter-moon windows.

- Turn right on Murdock Ave. The third house on your right is a pale-pink Arts and Crafts cottage from as early as 1920. Across 176th St., a classic Tudor with diamond-pane casement windows is further enhanced by its lush, exquisitely landscaped yard. It combines with the two superb properties opposite—one with red shutters and trim, the other projecting a two-story bay—for an unparalleled trio.

- Turn left on 177th St. Three houses in on your right, half-timbered dormers mimic the slopes of the main gable of a black-and-white house. Facing it, #112-40 was the home of Jackie Robinson during his historic tenure at second base for the Brooklyn Dodgers. Two years after breaking Major League Baseball's color barrier, Robinson moved from Brooklyn and resided here until he retired after the 1957 season.

- Turn right on 112th Ave., then right on 178th St. Singer Lena Horne lived at #112-45 in the 1940s and 1950s. Cross Murdock Ave. to an outstanding block that includes several 1920s Colonials: three of the first five on your right and three in a row on your left beginning with #114-33, with its Classical-style entrance of columns and side-lights. Above the door of #114-41 you will see a so-called swan-necked pediment.

- Make a left on 114th Rd. The first home on your left, with a shed dormer inset upstairs and trellises on both sides of the porch downstairs, was built in 1916 for Edwin H. Brown, the retired Manhattan lawyer who developed Addisleigh Park. Another Colonial is on the left past 178th Pl., with pink shutters. The houses across from it, identical when built in 1927, face each other and share a driveway.

- Turn right on 179th St. The first house on your right is—save for a ground-floor exten-sion—a dignified picture of symmetry, from the brick chimneys to the dormers with arched tops. Constructed in 1927, it's one of the few post-1920 homes on the block, and its garage occupies a separate lot. That's also the case with #114-91 across the street,. Both homes date to the late 1910s. The next two houses after that were part of Edwin H. Brown's first wave of development, as were the second and fifth houses on your right side. All of these have had some obvious refacing or addition.

- When you reach Linden Blvd., you're facing a Veterans Affairs (VA) nursing home. It replaced a 3,000-bed naval hospital, which had replaced a golf course during World War II. That's where Babe Ruth liked to golf. In 1931, when Ruth led the American League with 46 home runs and finished second in batting average (.373), a reporter asked about the highlight of his year; the slugger replied, "Shooting a 73 at St. Albans."

● Turn left on Linden Blvd., leaving the historic district and entering the commercial center of St. Albans. Murals celebrating local heritage are beneath the train trestle past 180th St.—famous residents painted on one side, early-20th-century life on the other. Farther along, visit the Maria Rose International Doll Museum at #187-11. Museum founder Naida Nelson Njoku acquired more than 500 dolls in her lifetime, and they are grouped according to their geographic origin in rooms dedicated to Africa and the Caribbean, the Americas and Antarctica, and Europe and Asia. Also on display are dolls of famous people ranging from Shirley Temple to Jacqueline Kennedy to Prince William and Kate Middleton. (The museum has been planning to relocate; if it's no longer here, you can visit its new location at the end of the tour.)

● Turn right on Everitt Pl. When you reach Baisley Blvd., it would be a short block to your left to Farmers Blvd., mentioned in a song by rapper LL Cool J (who grew up in St. Albans) on his best-selling album *Bigger and Deffer*—but make a right. Proceed on Baisley past the train and the VA facility. After the naval-hospital property was turned over to the VA in the 1970s, the agency gave half the land to the city for a park, which you enter across from 177th St. The building just inside Roy Wilkins Park on your right contains both a recreation center with an Olympic-size swimming pool and the Black Spectrum Theatre, which produces African American–themed plays and films and runs an extensive youth-outreach program. Guests of honor at its annual gala have included filmmaker Melvin Van Peebles and actors Ruby Dee and Ossie Davis.

● Follow the path across from the rec-center entrance. Stay to the left when it splits, walking with a pond on your right that may be overgrown with reeds.

● Continue on the path, or walk across the grass, to the running track and football field. Go to the right on the path encircling the track. You'll pass an enormous vegetable garden, one of two in the park cultivated by local residents. You'll see the other garden as you proceed around the track.

● Exit the park on Merrick Blvd. at Foch Blvd. There's a bus stop just to the right on Merrick, where you can get the Q5, Q84, or Q85 back to the subway in Jamaica. (If the doll museum has moved from Linden Blvd., it should be at 115-42 173rd St., a few blocks away: Turn right on Merrick Blvd. out of the park, then right on 116th Ave. and left on 173rd St.)

Note: See Walk 19's sidebar about Baisley Pond Park (page 154). One entrance to it is about 0.7 mile from where this walk ends. Walk west on Foch Blvd. from Merrick Blvd.

POINTS OF INTEREST

St. Albans Park Merrick Blvd. and Sayres Ave.

Maria Rose International Doll Museum & Cultural Center mariarose.biz, 187-11 Linden Blvd., 917-817-8653

Roy Wilkins Park Baisley Blvd. and Merrick Blvd.

Black Spectrum Theatre blackspectrum.com, Roy Wilkins Park, 718-723-1800

ROUTE SUMMARY

1. Walk east on Sayres Ave. from Merrick Blvd.
2. Turn right on Marne Pl.
3. Turn left at Adelaide Rd.
4. Make a right on 175th St.
5. Turn right on Murdock Ave.
6. Make a left on 174th St.
7. Make a left on Linden Blvd.
8. Turn left at 175th Pl.
9. Turn right on Murdock Ave.
10. Go left on 177th St.
11. Make a right on 112th Ave.
12. Turn right on 178th St.
13. Make a left on 114th Rd.
14. Make a right on 179th St.
15. Turn left on Linden Blvd.
16. Turn right on Everitt Pl.
17. Make a right on Baisley Blvd.
18. Enter Roy Wilkins Park at 177th St., and exit on Merrick Blvd.

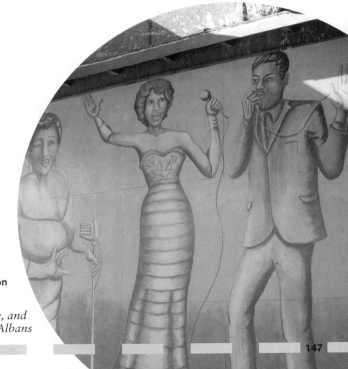

(From left) Ella Fitzgerald, Lena Horne, and Brook Benton . . . they all lived in St. Albans

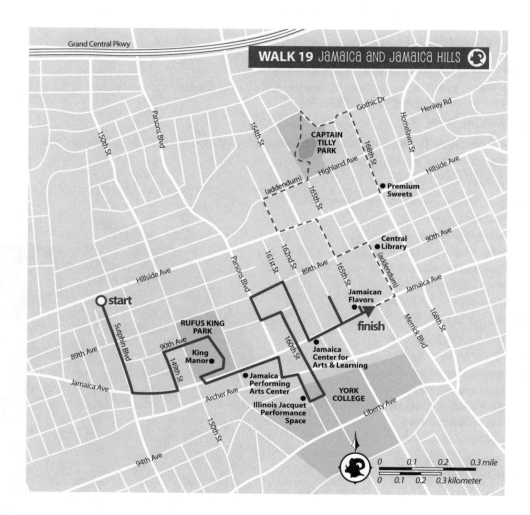

Grand Central Pkwy

150th St

Parsons Blvd

164th St

Gothic Dr

Henley Rd

Homelawn St

168th St

CAPTAIN TILLY PARK

Highland Ave

Hillside Ave

(addendum)

165th St

● Premium Sweets

Hillside Ave

Parsons Blvd

161st St

162nd St

89th Ave

90th Ave

Central Library
●

165th St

Jamaica Ave

(addendum)

○ **start**

Sutphin Blvd

RUFUS KING PARK

90th Ave

149th St

King Manor ●

160th St

Jamaican Flavors
●

finish ▶

Merrick Blvd

168th St

89th Ave

Jamaica Ave

Archer Ave

● Jamaica Center for Arts & Learning

● Jamaica Performing Arts Center

YORK COLLEGE

Illinois Jacquet Performance Space ●

Liberty Ave

150th St

94th Ave

0   0.1   0.2   0.3 mile

0   0.1   0.2   0.3 kilometer

19 JAMAICA AND JAMAICA HILLS: AT THE CROSSROADS

BOUNDARIES: Gothic Dr., 168th St., York College, Sutphin Blvd.
DISTANCE: 2.4 or 3.8 miles, depending on route chosen
SUBWAY: F to Sutphin Blvd.

George Washington slept here. Really. "A pretty good and decent house," Washington wrote in his diary about the Jamaica lodgings on his post-Revolution salutatory tour of Long Island in April 1790. The inn where he stayed stood at Jamaica Ave. and Parsons Blvd. until 1906. Though it's gone, the number of surviving historic structures is impressive, especially considering all the people, construction, and transportation—from horse-drawn carts to the JFK AirTrain—that have come through Jamaica since it was chartered in the 1650s. Incorporated as a village in 1814 and served by the Long Island Rail Road since 1834, Jamaica was selected as county seat of Queens because it was located approximately halfway between the East River (that is, Manhattan) and the Suffolk County line (the eastern boundary of Queens before it was incorporated into NYC in 1898). The large neighborhood extends in all directions beyond the bounds of this walk, which focuses on downtown Jamaica, a bustling district where everyone from a Founding Father of our country to a founding father of hip-hop has left a mark.

● Use the Sutphin Blvd. and Hillside Ave. southside exit from the subway, and proceed straight ahead on Sutphin Blvd. The courthouse on your left after 88th Ave. was a New Deal project. Round benches on the plaza are engraved with the names of Queens communities, and bronze artwork outside the building includes the *Wheel of Justice* plaza centerpiece and sculpted panels around the arched doorways that depict people and objects associated with law throughout world history (look for Confucius, Muhammad, and Hammurabi, among others). The Supreme Court interior—with black marble columns and vaulted ceilings—is worth seeing too, and you're welcome to go inside on workdays. Once you are through the security checkpoint, head to the rear of the building, where *Constitutional Law* and *Mosaic Law* paintings hang above a marble staircase.

- Back on Sutphin Blvd., take note of the message inscribed on the bank to your right as you approach Jamaica Ave. This fine example of Moderne architecture, constructed in 1939 for the Jamaica Savings Bank, has been designated a landmark. Business hours permitting, go inside to see what Jamaica looked like in 1840, according to a mural behind the tellers.

- With your back to the bank, go left on Jamaica Ave.

- Turn left on 149th St., then right on 90th Ave. You can see on the street signs that it's also named Rufus King Ave., and it takes you right into a park also named for him. King was a signer of the Constitution, New York's first US senator, and an ambassador to Britain. This park comprises 11 of the 90 acres he purchased in Jamaica in 1805. To go straight to his house (open Thursday–Sunday), follow the path on the right inside the park, but you may wish to meander through the tree- and bench-filled park before or after visiting King Manor. Its excellent docent-led tour includes such highlights as the library where King, an avid writer and reader, spent most of his waking time; an upstairs guest room where John Quincy Adams spent the night; and the remnant of a French flag gifted by General Marquis de Lafayette. The guide can also show you a drawing of a noose with King's name hanging from it—one of many death threats he received due to his staunch abolitionism. John Alsop King, Rufus's son, owned the house after his father and served as a congressman and governor.

- Exit the park on Jamaica Ave. near 150th St., and go to your left. Looking at King Manor from the sidewalk, you can read the preamble to the Constitution on the front gate. On the other side of the avenue, the walls of the Family Court building (designed by I. M. Pei's firm) bear a tribute to Thurgood Marshall, the trailblazing Supreme Court justice. Across 153rd St., the former First Reformed Church has been converted to the Jamaica Performing Arts Center, its Romanesque magnificence and stained glass windows intact. This 1859 building was the third church constructed for First Reformed, founded as a Dutch-speaking congregation in 1702; its previous homes are commemorated in the wedge-shaped tablet between the two front doors.

- Cross back to the north side of the avenue. Half a block east of 153rd, the 1862 brownstone Gothic structure is home to Grace Episcopal, the oldest Episcopal congregation on Long Island and second oldest in New York State (after Manhattan's

Trinity Church). This building, like First Reformed's, has been awarded landmark status. Among the long-ago residents of Jamaica buried in the churchyard are Rufus and John Alsop King, to your left when facing the church.

● Make a right on Parsons Blvd.

● Turn left on Archer Ave., then pass through the York College gates under the train tracks. On your right is historic Prospect Cemetery, where upward of 3,000 people were laid to rest starting in the 1660s. Many graves have lost their markers, but family names include Van Wyck, Brinkerhoff, and Sutphin, all of whom have local roads named for them. The cemetery is open only for occasional tours, usually run by the Prospect Cemetery Association, which maintains it. The group was involved in restoring the cemetery's chapel, now a venue of York College's Jazz Forum. Named the Chapel of the Sisters when it was built in 1857 by a businessman who'd lost three young daughters (all buried in Prospect), it was renamed the Illinois Jacquet Performance Space in honor of the well-known jazz saxophonist, a longtime resident of nearby St. Albans (see Walk 18). The college, opened in 1967, is part of the City University of New York. Its unique departments include an Aviation Institute, training students for management positions in an industry that employs many in Queens; the Black American Heritage Foundation, which includes a Music History Archive of documents, recordings, and personal possessions from professional musicians; and the Northeast Regional Laboratory of the Food and Drug Administration.

● Go on the path across the way from the cemetery, which takes you to

Jamaica Ave. near Union Hall St.

160th St. En route, you can see how a new building was added on to St. Monica's bell tower—all that remained of the 1856 church after a storm felled it in the 1990s. One of Long Island's oldest Catholic congregations, St. Monica's had an altar boy in the 1940s named Mario Cuomo, who grew up to be a governor of New York and the father of a governor of New York.

● Proceed north on 160th St., across Archer and Jamaica Aves. Two landmarks are located within one block on your right. First, the stainless steel home of the Jamaica Business Resource Center (JBRC) was built for a nightclub called La Casina in a Streamline Moderne style most commonly deployed on roadside buildings like hotels, diners, and bus terminals. La Casina went out of business after just a few years, and the building later was used as a bra and swimsuit factory. It was rescued from severe neglect by the Greater Jamaica Development Corp. (GJDC), which helped establish the JBRC as the pilot location of a federal small-business initiative. The development agency is headquartered in the Art Deco landmark at the end of the block, built for a mortgage firm in the late 1920s and now housing a variety of government and nonprofit offices. Its polychromatic terra-cotta panels were sculpted by an artist who also worked on Radio City Music Hall.

● Turn left on 90th Ave.

● At Parsons Blvd., take a look at Grace Episcopal's 1912 parish house across on the left, but turn right. Next to a white-steepled church, the building resembling a Renaissance palace is having its third life: First it was a library, then a courthouse, and now it's part of Moda, a LEED-certified residential building with on-site shopping and an allotment of apartments for low-income households. While the Family Court that took over the building in 1970 left its name inscribed, there are more-artistic reminders of the library for which it was built in the late 1920s: Look on the sides of the lamppost pedestals for a book, an owl, and a lamp, all symbols of wisdom. Prefer your ornamentation faith-based? Check out the massive Presentation of the Blessed Virgin Mary Church, on your right at 89th Ave. This parish was composed of German immigrants when founded in the 1880s.

● Go to the right on 89th Ave. The buildings facing each other across 161st St. are particularly attractive at their tops, with arched dormer windows to your left and domes to your right.

- Turn right on 161st St. Another landmark representing another architectural style stands on your left at #89-31, the neo-Georgian Chamber of Commerce building. It's opposite the Title Guarantee building you saw from 160th St., which has fewer doorway dragons than this side! Proceed to Jamaica Ave. and look across for an excellent view of Jamaica's Financial Row. The two buildings with wrought iron balconies date to 1898 and are landmarks. They and their 1920s neighbors to the right were all built for financial and real estate outfits, but none is currently used for its original purpose. Directly across from 161st St., the former Jamaica Savings Bank headquarters is considered the Beaux Arts masterpiece of Queens. Note the beehive, a symbol of thrift often found on old banks, beneath the upper balcony. While the beautiful bank has stood vacant for years, the Register of Title and Deeds building to the left of it has been repurposed as the Jamaica Center for Arts & Learning (JCAL). Inside its Italian Renaissance home, JCAL has a theater, art gallery, and art and music studios.

- Cross Jamaica Ave. and go to your left. The cast-iron clock at the corner is yet another official landmark, a turn-of-the-century relic of an age when stores would invest in advertising like this—the name of the business that installed the clock would encircle the clockface, as JAMAICA CENTER does now—and many people depended on these clocks for the time because they didn't own wristwatches (let alone cell phones). See the plaques on the Union Hall St. side of the corner building for more about the clock as well as a lost church of colonial Jamaica.

  Proceeding along Jamaica Ave., note the PLAUT BROS name atop #162-11. Plaut's was an early department store, succeeded as the prime shopping destination of Jamaica by Gertz just across the street. The Gertz department store occupied #162-10 from the 1920s until 1980. Coincidentally, another local retail giant of its era was not only located right next door but had a rhyming name, Kurtz. The six-story building at the corner of Guy R. Brewer Blvd. was constructed exclusively for the Kurtz furniture store. Look at the building on its Brewer Blvd. side, where signs shouldn't obscure the Art Deco detail that earned it landmark status. While still in front of the store, cross Jamaica Ave. for an optimal view of the building just to the east, which features violin medallions above its windows. At 163rd St., look across to the retail mishmash that resides in the grandeur of the former Merrick movie house.

- Make a left onto 164th St. First Presbyterian Church, on your left, was erected a block away on Jamaica Ave. in 1813. It was placed on a flatbed of logs and pulled by mules

BaISLeY POND ParK

About 2 miles south of downtown Jamaica, Baisley Pond Park centers on a 30-acre watery habitat for lily pads, turtles, ducks, and geese. You might even see a heron, egret, or bullfrog. Toward its north end, the pond teems with reeds. Created when 18th-century farmers dammed streams to power their grain mill, Baisley Pond was later used as a reservoir for the city of Brooklyn. Municipal workers dredging it in the 1850s unearthed five molar teeth and fragments of bone and tusk—the 10,000-year-old remains of a mastodon. This incredible prehistoric discovery is commemorated in one of the park's playgrounds, which holds a life-size mastodon statue for kids to climb on.

To go to the park after the Jamaica walk, take the Q6 (bound for JFK Airport) from the bus terminal on Merrick Blvd. across from the Central Library; if you're making a separate trip, take the Q6 from the E or F Sutphin Blvd. station. For the mastodon and pond, get off the bus on Sutphin Blvd. at Rockaway Blvd. and enter the park at their northeast intersection, where stone pillars flank a path. Go straight ahead on the bench-lined path toward the flagpole, but look to your left to see the mastodon across a field. Follow the path to the World War I memorial behind the flagpole, then go to your right for the path around the pond. Proceed counterclockwise to a terrace at the water's edge, with benches and frog sculptures, then continue around the pond. The 110-acre park also has facilities for almost every sport: tennis, basketball, cricket, handball, baseball, track, football, you name it. There's even a checkers-and-chess pavilion south of Rockaway Blvd. On the north side of the boulevard, summer concerts are held in a large open field.

to this site in 1920, to escape the noise from the increasingly busy avenue. Organized in 1662 and believed to be the oldest US Presbyterian congregation in existence, it was an original benefactor of Presbyterian-founded Princeton University. Next to the church, set back from the sidewalk, is a cute manse built in the 1830s and resuscitated after decades of abandonment for educational use.

● Return to Jamaica Ave. from the church, and turn left. Want to enjoy some Jamaican food while you're in Jamaica, even though the neighborhood's name has nothing to do with the Caribbean island? It's still a prominent cuisine locally, as the area has a significant West Indian population. Just off the avenue to your left, along the 165th St. pedestrian mall, buy a patty from Jamaican Flavors. *This* Jamaica, meanwhile, came from an Anglicization of either the name of a local tribe or a native word for *beaver,* originally transcribed as *yamecah* or *jameco.* Back on the avenue, a half block farther, you can't miss one of the most extraordinary structures in all of New York, the Valencia theater. Its marquee bears the name of the subsequent occupant, the Tabernacle of Prayer. Opened in 1929 as a 3,500-seat flagship of the Loew's movie-theater chain, the Valencia represents an architectural style with a name as elaborate as the decor: Churrigueresque, a variant of Spanish Baroque. Behind this facade of nautical, agricultural, and celestial figures are an even more lavish lobby and auditorium, which the church—to whom Loew's donated the building—has spent more than $1 million maintaining. Amazingly, during the theater's 50 years in business, passersby on the street could barely see it—an elevated train ran along Jamaica Ave. until 1980.

● On the same side of the avenue, any of the buses that stop at 165th St. connect to the E, J, and Z train. Or continue on to Jamaica Hills.

aDDeNDUM

● Turn left from Jamaica Ave. onto Merrick Blvd. At #90-10 was the 24/7 recording studio, where rap legend Jam Master Jay of Run-DMC was shot to death in October 2002. (A tribute to the group's deejay, born Jason Mizell, is found not where he died but where he lived: Hollis, the neighborhood just east of Jamaica, where he's honored in a mural on 205th St.) Farther down the block on your right is the Central Library of the Queens system. It owns so many books that about half of them are stored underground and retrieved on request. The building also contains a 100-computer Cyber Center and interactive science-themed exhibits for children. The library has an exchange program with a Shanghai library, and it holds a premier collection of historical documents and artifacts related to Queens.

- Turn left on 89th Ave.

- Turn right on 164th St. The stately post office on your left is listed on the National Register of Historic Places.

- Make a left on Hillside Ave. The school on your left between 163rd and 162nd Sts. has dormers you don't see very often—they're called (for obvious reasons) "witch's hats" and are merely the crowning detail of this Flemish Revival landmark. It is a rare Queens product of Gilded Age architect William Tubby, who designed many mansions and institutional buildings in Brooklyn. Upon its completion in 1896, this building housed primary and secondary schools, but by 1909, the population had grown so much that younger grades were moved elsewhere and this became known as Jamaica High School. Within 20 years, it too was insufficiently sized, and another Jamaica High School (which you will see shortly) was built. It's now an alternative high school.

- Turn right on 162nd St., crossing into Jamaica Hills north of Hillside Ave.

- Make a right on Highland Ave. At 165th St., go into Captain Tilly Park, an oasis that seems hidden despite its proximity to the business district. Following the path, watch on your left for a granite monument honoring United Spanish War Veterans. Additional memorials sit beneath the flagpole, including an evocative bronze relief that, interestingly, heads off any possible rumors about its composition in its engraving. Captain Tilly, who was killed in the Philippines, was a son in the family that used to own this land. It later was acquired by the Highland Park Society, who raised ducks and geese on a pond fed by underground springs. Enjoy the sights and sounds of Goose Pond, walking in either direction on the path around it and detouring, if you'd like, onto the woodsy path off to the left. When you're on the other side of the pond, follow the path between the playground and the water.

● Exit the park on curvy Gothic Dr. Look to your left at a pale blue house with a chimney painted to match. That shade of blue in this area usually signals property owned by followers of Sri Chinmoy, the controversial late guru who built his spiritual center/empire/cult (depends on whose stories you believe) in Jamaica Hills.

● Make a right on Gothic Dr., walking beside the expansive grounds of the second Jamaica High School. The school switched to this building from the one on Hillside Ave. in 1927, and like its predecessor, it's been landmarked. Its Georgian Revival style, a traditional choice for American civic buildings, was an assimilating tactic intended to benefit the largely immigrant student body. Its front doors, crowned by fanlights, are made of bronze and set within archways beneath the columns. Facing out from the rock-faced double staircase opposite 167th St. is a dramatic memorial to alumni who died in World War II, their names flanking the David-like figure. Jamaica High's famous alumni include *Godfather* director Francis Ford Coppola, feminist writer Letty Cottin Pogrebin, 1968 Olympic long-jump champion Bob Beamon, and Watergate conspirator John Mitchell.

● Go one more block on Gothic to 168th St., and turn right. You see the Al-Mamoor mosque well before you're in front of it. Started in a basement in 1976, it has brought many South Asians into the neighborhood. A block and a half farther, grab a South Asian snack from Premium Sweets, to the left on Hillside Ave. The entrance to the F train is at the corner.

World War II memorial on the high school grounds

POINTS OF INTEREST

Rufus King Park 90th Ave. and 150th St.

King Manor kingmanor.org, 150-03 Jamaica Ave., 718-206-0545

Jamaica Performing Arts Center jamaica-performingartscenter.org,
153-10 Jamaica Ave., 718-618-6170

Illinois Jacquet Performance Space jazzatthechapel.org, 94-15 159th St.

York College york.cuny.edu, 94-20 Guy R. Brewer Blvd., 718-262-2000

Jamaica Center for Arts & Learning jcal.org, 161-04 Jamaica Ave., 718-658-7400

Jamaican Flavors jamaicanflavors.com, 164-17B Jamaica Ave., 718-526-2228

ADDENDUM POINTS OF INTEREST

Central Library queenslibrary.org/central-library, 89-11 Merrick Blvd., 718-990-0700

Captain Tilly Park Highland Ave. and 165th St.

Premium Sweets 168-03 Hillside Ave., 718-739-6000

route summary

1. Walk south on Sutphin Blvd. from Hillside Ave.
2. Turn left on Jamaica Ave.
3. Make a left on 149th St.
4. Turn right on 90th Ave. and enter Rufus King Park.
5. Exit the park on Jamaica Ave. (near 150th St.), and walk east.
6. Turn right on Parsons Blvd.
7. Make a left on Archer Ave.
8. Turn right into the York College campus, using a path to head east.
9. Go left on 160th St.
10. Make a left on 90th Ave.
11. Make a right on Parsons Blvd.
12. Turn right on 89th Ave.
13. Make a right on 161st St.
14. Make a left on Jamaica Ave.
15. Turn left on 164th St.
16. Return to Jamaica Ave. and make a left.

addendum

17. Make a left on Merrick Blvd.
18. Go left on 89th Ave.
19. Turn right on 164th St.
20. Turn left on Hillside Ave.
21. Turn right on 162nd St.
22. Make a right on Highland Ave.
23. Enter Captain Tilly Park at 165th St.
24. Exit the park on Gothic Dr. and make a right.
25. Go right on 168th St. to Hillside Ave.

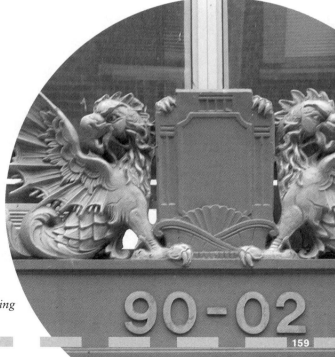

Above the door of the Title Guarantee building

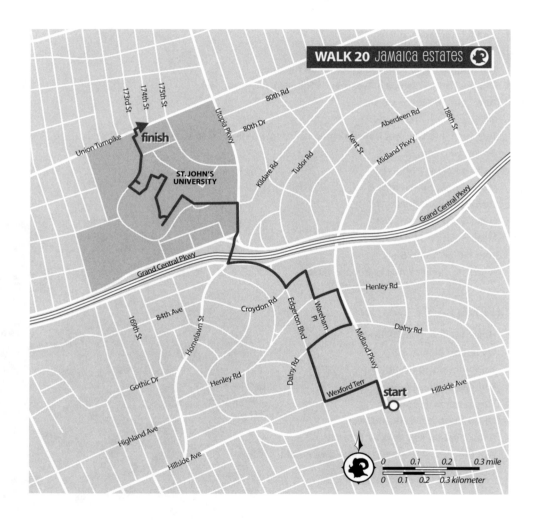

173rd St

174th St

175th St

80th Rd

Utopia Pkwy

80th Dr

Aberdeen Rd

Kent St

Midland Pkwy

188th St

finish

Union Turnpike

ST. JOHN'S UNIVERSITY

Kildare Rd

Tudor Rd

Grand Central Pkwy

Grand Central Pkwy

Henley Rd

Croydon Rd

Edgerton Blvd

Wareham Pl

Dalny Rd

84th Ave

169th St

Homelawn St

Midland Pkwy

Dalny Rd

Gothic Dr

Henley Rd

Dalny Rd

Wexford Terr

start

Hillside Ave

Highland Ave

Hillside Ave

0   0.1   0.2   0.3 mile

0   0.1   0.2   0.3 kilometer

20 Jamaica Estates: Luxe Living and the College Life

BOUNDARIES: Union Tpke., Midland Pkwy., Hillside Ave., 173rd St.
DISTANCE: 2.1 miles
SUBWAY: F to 179th St.

A residential park. Nice idea, isn't it? That's what the developers of Jamaica Estates had in mind when they began to transform forested highlands north of Jamaica into a residential community in 1907. It would have the natural beauty of a park, but you could live there. To effect the parklike setting, the developers respected the contours of the land: Hills were not leveled, and no rectangular street grid was forced through. Jamaica Estates would have winding roads, like park drives—with British names for extra prestige. The Jamaica Estates Company made beauty and exclusivity priorities for their development rather than maximizing profitability per acre . . . which may have had something to do with the firm going bankrupt after just over a decade in business. It was left to a homeowners' association to preserve its vision, and while apartment houses were eventually built in Jamaica Estates, much of it has kept to the original plan for high-quality freestanding homes, and the neighborhood remains a leafy Tudor enclave.

● Use the Midland Pkwy. exit from the subway on the north side of Hillside Ave., which separates Jamaica Estates from Jamaica. On the median mall is the Jamaica Estates gatehouse, akin to something you might see at the entry to an English manor. Providing a formal entrance to the community since the beginning, it was designed by John J. Petit, architect of San Francisco's Hearst Building and the Coney Island amusement park Dreamland. It was originally complemented by a stone lodge, also designed by Petit, where the Midland Gardens apartments now stand. Across the parkway from Midland Gardens is a house with a Japanese lantern and rock garden.

● Turn left on Wexford Terr. The Catholic Church has a significant presence in this corner of Jamaica Estates. The Paulist Fathers are headquartered on Midland Pkwy., and the large property to your right belongs to the Passionist Order. Up the hill across

HOLLISWOOD AND THE OTHER HOLLISES

Like Jamaica Estates? Then check out its next-door neighbor Holliswood. It was developed separately but also resembles a residential park, with curvy roads, abundant foliage, and commodious lawns. The border between the two communities is 188th St. Holliswood's housing stock is younger on average but encompasses both classic and contemporary styles. On Santiago St., houses sit atop hills and low stone walls enclose some yards. Palo Alto St. is worth seeing for its sheer variety. (Also on this street, a yeshiva is across from a Sikh temple.) On Nero Ave. around Palermo and Sancho Sts., marvel at the height of the trees—and some picture-perfect landscaping. The neighborhood's winding layout makes it easy to wander. Developer Frederick W. Dunton designed looping roads and gave them names containing the letter *o* because, as an astrology buff, he had a circular affinity. The Holliswood road Epsom Course used to be a trot-racing oval that Dunton built.

You'll also want to walk Foothill Ave. off of 191st St. On the north side, a few extravagant homes are situated at extravagant elevations. East of 193rd St., Foothill Ave. is brick-paved and offers terrific views between the houses.

Dunton developed another nice residential community, Hollis Park Gardens, south of Holliswood. On the south side of Hillside Ave. (the boundary between the neighborhoods), brick gateposts bear an entwined HPG monogram sculpted in relief, as well as the original street names, like Fairmount Ave. for 195th St. For a sampling, take 195th Pl. (Restwood Ave. per the gatepost) from Hillside Ave., then turn right on 90th Ave. From there, go left down any street to Jamaica Ave.—the border with Hollis proper. The name Hollis came from the New Hampshire town where Dunton grew up. Affluent Hollis Hills is northwest of Holliswood.

In Hollis Park Gardens

Edgerton Blvd. is Mary Louis Academy, a Catholic girls' high school founded by nuns in the 1930s.

● Turn right on Edgerton Blvd. Nuns who teach at Mary Louis live in the Spanish Mission–style convent on your left. The building next to it with arched doorways was one of the neighborhood's early mansions, built in 1911. Across the street, another private estate was turned over to the Passionist Order. For its parish, established in 1923 by the bishop of Brooklyn (a diocese that includes Queens), the Passionists acquired the home of Michael Degnon, a contractor—and devout Catholic—whose firm built part of the NYC subway, as well as the streets, sewers, and utilities systems of Jamaica Estates. The congregation held its first services in Degnon's former mansion, which would be demolished when the retreat house was enlarged around 1950.

Continuing up Edgerton, you will start to see some of the dignified residences of Jamaica Estates. The one near the end of the block on your left houses a sort of Hindu counterpart to the Passionist retreat center: an ashram devoted to the teachings of early-20th-century guru Sri Ramana Maharsh and established by a follower named Arunachala, who moved it here from the East Village in the 1980s.

● Turn right on Dalny Rd., where even the bay window of the fairy-tale Tudor on your left has a slate roof. Downhill on your right is Immaculate Conception School, opened by the Passionists in 1938. The parish's convent is next to the school on Midland Pkwy.

● Turn left on Midland Pkwy., the central boulevard of Jamaica Estates. The interesting mix of religious organizations based in the neighborhood includes the synagogue on your left at #85-34, Bene Naharayim, a congregation of Iraqi Jews. (Jamaica Estates also has a synagogue for Afghan Jews.)

● Turn left on Henley Rd. The second house on your right is a good representation of what was envisioned for Jamaica Estates—exceptional, Tudor-influenced residences on verdant lots—and its petite, distinctly shaped windows in the attic and entry vestibule enhance its character.

● Make a right on Wareham Pl., a block where you can see homes that fulfilled the original concept for Jamaica Estates and more-modern replacements. Facing you at Croydon Rd. is a, shall we say, Shakespearean-nautical hybrid, as pretty as it is unique.

- Make a left on Croydon Rd. and then the first right, which is Edgerton Blvd. Highlights include the stone castle tower of a half-timbered house and its green-and-white Colonial neighbor.

- Go to the left at the traffic island, which puts you on the Grand Central Pkwy. service road. When the highway was constructed in the 1930s (replacing a boulevard called Doncaster), the homeowners' association jumped into action to keep the road noncommercial.

- Make a right at the crosswalk at Homelawn St., and follow the sidewalk through the underpass. On the other side, you will be on Utopia Pkwy.

- Proceed to the entrance to the St. John's University campus opposite Kildare Rd. This was the site of the Hillcrest Golf Club, created in the design for Jamaica Estates. St. John's, a Catholic university founded in Brooklyn in 1870, has had its main campus here since the 1950s. It is probably best known for its men's basketball team, which ranks in the top 10 in all-time NCAA victories and made the playoffs all 24 seasons Lou Carnesecca was coach.

- Walk straight ahead on the main campus road. To your right is the law school, whose bronze facade sculpture reinterprets the scales of justice: Divine law (the Ten Commandments) at the base balances codified law and common law. Codified law is on the left, with cuneiform and the standing figure representing Hammurabi and his code. The oak tree, meanwhile, is a traditional symbol of the Magna Carta, shaper of American law—the 13 stars around the tree a stand-in for the United States and its 13 original colonies.

- Stepping onto the quad, or Great Lawn in St. John's parlance, you have St. John Hall, the oldest building on campus, on your right. Turn onto the Founders Ln. path in front of it, which takes you to the Celtic cross monument. Even the a-religious may appreciate its theme of "peace and harmony within the human family" and the sculpting on the cross. Proceed on the path to the chapel. The university had intended to build a freestanding church ever since it opened its Queens campus, but it took half a century—and the largesse of a law-school alumnus—for the plan to be realized. Do go inside if you can. The mosaics encircling the foyer, which illustrate Vincentian heritage, were handcrafted in Florence, Italy. In the sanctuary, stained glass windows burst with color, water cascades down a 9/11 memorial to the left, and a bronze statue of the chapel's namesake, Thomas More (the patron saint of lawyers), stands beneath the organ pipes. Leave the church via the side door next to the vocation director's office, and walk through its garden and back to the Great Lawn. Continue around, passing St. Augustine Hall (the large central building) on your way to a fountain terrace.

- Walk through the covered passageway between the welcome center and registrar's office to a landing facing a tower that holds a golden torch. You're also overlooking Sun Yat Sen Memorial Hall, built for the Asian-studies department and modeled on an ancient Chinese palace. Go down the stairs and make a left at the fountain on Loughlin Ln.

- Turn right on St. Albert Way and continue to the front entrance of the "palace," flanked by lion statues. The art gallery inside is open every day except Sunday and Monday. If it's closed, at least look inside the doorway at an oversize statue of Confucius. Opposite the pagoda is the D'Angelo Center, a recent (2009) addition to the campus housing the student union. Walk toward its tower, then go past it and head downhill to a sidewalk clock, which bears the same name as the field house next to it. Donald L. Taffner, the late alumnus who endowed the field house, was an Emmy-winning producer who distributed British series such as *The Benny Hill Show* and *Rumpole of the Bailey* for American TV. The university's basketball arena and football stadium are to your right, but use the staircase beside the Taffner clock to exit the campus. Down the steps, walk past the running track and tennis courts to reach Union Tpke.

- Cross Union Tpke. at 173rd St. and go to the right, where you can get the Q46 bus to the E or F train in Kew Gardens.

POINTS OF INTEREST

St. John's University stjohns.edu, 8000 Utopia Pkwy., 718-990-2000

Dr. M. T. Geoffrey Yeh Art Gallery tinyurl.com/yehgallery, Sun Yat Sen Memorial Hall, St. John's University, 718-990-7476

route summary

1. Walk north on Midland Pkwy. from Hillside Ave.
2. Turn left on Wexford Terr.
3. Turn right on Edgerton Blvd.
4. Make a right on Dalny Rd.
5. Make a left on Midland Pkwy.
6. Turn left on Henley Rd.
7. Go right on Wareham Pl.
8. Go left on Croydon Rd.
9. Turn right on Edgerton Blvd.
10. Make a left on Grand Central Pkwy. service road.
11. Turn right on Homelawn St., which becomes Utopia Pkwy.
12. Turn left at Kildare Rd.
13. Walk through St. John's campus.
14. Exit at Union Tpke. and 173rd St.

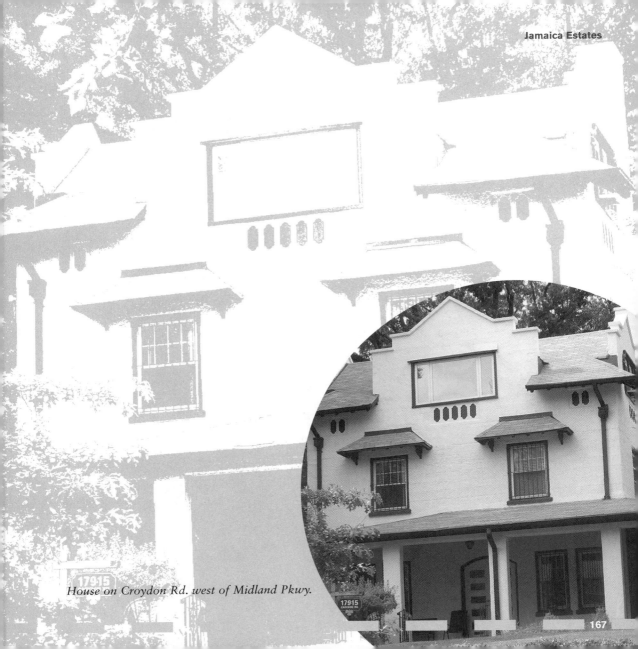

House on Croydon Rd. west of Midland Pkwy.

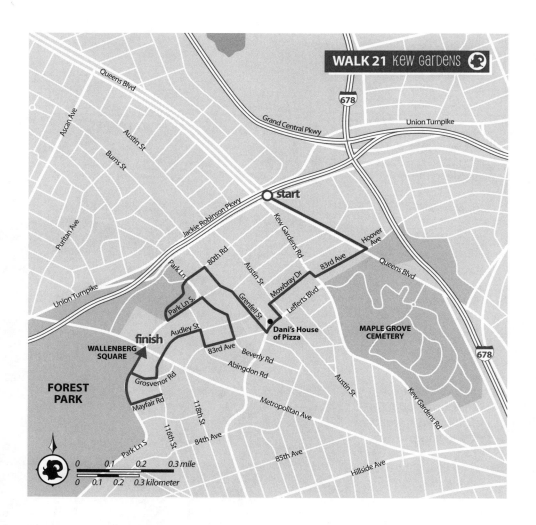

678

Queens Blvd

Ascan Ave

Austin St

Burns St

Grand Central Pkwy

Union Turnpike

Puritan Ave

Jackie Robinson Pkwy

start

Kew Gardens Rd

Hoover Ave

Park Ln

80th Rd

Austin St

83rd Ave

Queens Blvd

Union Turnpike

Park Ln S.

Grenfell St

Mowbray Dr

Lefferts Blvd

finish

Audley St

Dani's House of Pizza

MAPLE GROVE CEMETERY

WALLENBERG SQUARE

83rd Ave

Beverly Rd

Grosvenor Rd

Abingdon Rd

Austin St

FOREST PARK

Mayfair Rd

118th St

Metropolitan Ave

Kew Gardens Rd

678

Park Ln S

116th St

84th Ave

85th Ave

Hillside Ave

0   0.1   0.2   0.3 mile
0   0.1   0.2   0.3 kilometer

21 Kew Gardens: Tudor Suburb in the City

BOUNDARIES: Queens Blvd., Mayfair Rd., Park Ln. S., 80th Rd.
DISTANCE: 2.5 miles, plus optional 1.25-mile nature walk
SUBWAY: E or F to Kew Gardens–Union Tpke.

The word *suburb* had a different meaning when American cities started growing dramatically in the early 20th century. It used to refer to areas removed geographically from the busy urban center but not necessarily outside the city limits. Walking distance to shops, other homes, and public transit was one of the urban qualities retained for early suburbs; the noise and crowdedness, along with lack of fresh air and greenery, were the urban characteristics they eschewed. Kew Gardens was created as one of these suburbs. Established by attorney Alrick Man in 1910, Kew Gardens got its name from a place in Britain; street names and Tudor half-timbering were also borrowed from the English. Other styles entered the mix to produce an assortment of lovely houses, and despite some undesirable modifications and replacements in recent years, the ideal of attractive suburban living within a half-hour commute of midtown perseveres in Kew Gardens.

● In the subway station, follow exit signs for 80th Rd. and Union Tpke. on the north side of Queens Blvd. When you reach the sidewalk, the high-rise office tower you see across Queens Blvd. gives a misleading first impression of Kew Gardens. It was built on the site of the Kew Gardens Inn, one of two hotels included in the neighborhood's original layout; the inn was converted in the 1940s into a hospital, later demolished.

● As you walk east on Queens Blvd. (with its roadway on your right), look across at the taller brick building, Kew Bolmer—you can see the name above the arch between storefronts. This was Kew Gardens' first apartment building, opened in 1915; more than 20 of them would be erected in the neighborhood by 1939.

Decades after the residential community of Kew Gardens was developed, the area became a civic center for Queens when the borough government and county courthouse were relocated here. On your left, you'll approach an extremely long building that looks like it belongs on a college campus. This is Queens Borough Hall, admittedly no match for the elegant domed borough and city halls of Brooklyn and

THE GARDEN CEMETERY OF KEW GARDENS

Maple Grove Cemetery opened in 1875 while Richmond Hill, the community south of Kew Gardens, was being developed. Albon Platt Man and Alrick Man, the father and son who created those two garden suburbs, are among the distinguished New Yorkers interred at Maple Grove. Celebrities buried there include jazz singer Jimmy Rushing, showman and composer Vincent Youmans ("Tea for Two"), and recording artist LaVern Baker, a member of the Rock & Roll Hall of Fame. The cemetery also contains some fine statuary: kindly-faced angels, human figures bearing symbolic objects, and dramatically sculpted tableaux.

Maple Grove comes out of the Victorian era's rural cemetery tradition, beautifully landscaped with ponds, trees, and gentle hills. There were not many public parks in those days, so people visited cemeteries for nature outings. Maple Grove even had its own train station until the Long Island Rail Road established a stop for Kew Gardens.

Enter on Kew Gardens Rd. at Lefferts Blvd. where the original Queen Anne–style administration building stands. Its stone came from Maple Grove's own (now-defunct) quarry. Architect James E. Ware received $100 and a cemetery plot for 12 as payment for designing the building. This compact older part of the cemetery is easy to wander through on your own. Markers point you to graves and monuments with "story stones," which illuminate a chapter in Maple Grove history or accomplishments of a "resident."

Going east, look for the Presidential Circle, the 9/11 memorial, and the lake. In the cemetery's modern administrative center, artifacts related to the cemetery and its notable interred are on display. A group called the Friends of Maple Grove sponsors concerts, walking tours, and interpretive events to raise awareness of its heritage and the lives of those laid to rest here.

Manhattan, which predate this early-1940s building by more than a century. Yet here's an achievement they can't claim: This borough hall holds the offices of the Queens borough president, a position that's been held by a woman since the mid-1980s.

- To the left of the entrance, visit the Veterans Memorial Garden. While this pleasant oasis was intended, obviously, as a somber place, on weekdays it's often filled with smiling couples who just got married in Queens Borough Hall and are taking their wedding photos. On the other side of the entry plaza, look on the ground for the Queens tricentennial time capsule.

  The old subway car on the lawn near 82nd Ave. (a tourist-information center) is a Redbird, the type of car used on Queens' 7 line until 2003. These were the last trains where riders could be straphangers (handrails have superseded straps), and while everyone knows them these days as Redbirds, they were not painted that color until the 1980s as part of the MTA's graffiti cleanup.

- Cross 82nd Ave. to survey the other behemoth of bureaucracy on this strip, the Queens County Criminal Courts Building. It's a bland midcentury construction, though its kinetic sculpture and the reliefs above doors on the east and west ends offer some enhancement.

- Make a right at Hoover Ave., which becomes 83rd Ave. as you cross Queens Blvd. Walk uphill to Kew Gardens Rd. and look across it to your left at the First Church of Kew Gardens, erected in the 1920s and designed by Hobart Upjohn, whose father and grandfather (both named Richard) were preeminent church architects of the 19th century. Across from the church is Maple Grove Cemetery, which you can detour into (see sidebar for details).

- Turn right from 83rd Ave. onto Kew Gardens Rd., coming around P.S. 99.

- Turn left in front of the school onto Mowbray Dr. When the city imposed its street numbering system on Kew Gardens, Mowbray Pl. was to become 82nd Dr. Every family on the block signed a petition for the mayor objecting to the change. They got to keep Mowbray but not Place because, per the Queens street grid, only roads and drives run parallel to avenues; places and lanes go with streets. Walking down Mowbray, you can understand the residents' pride. These impressive homes represent a variety of styles, including the Dutch Colonial that was fashionable in their era. Some accounts have Charlie Chaplin living in the Arts and Crafts–style house at #105 in its early years, but more likely it belonged to his manager, Samuel Hadley.

Upon reaching Austin St., look at the enigmatic ornamentation, complete with Latin adages, on the Mowbray building on your left. This was the tallest apartment house in Queens when it opened in the mid-1920s, boasting such state-of-the-art amenities as electric elevators and iceless refrigerators. There was a time later on when those living here were regarded as the worst neighbors in the world—if the initial news reports about the murder of Kitty Genovese are to be believed. Genovese was repeatedly stabbed outside her home in March 1964 while, it was reported in the weeks that followed, 38 neighbors witnessed the attack but did nothing to help. Genovese's home was the top floor of the building across Austin, next to the railroad station. To this day, a dispute persists over how many people heard or saw the crime, but the incident is still invoked in reference to public apathy.

● Cross Austin St., walk through the train station's small parking lot, and make a left, heading toward the staircase. Looking to your right, you can see that Lefferts Blvd. spans the Long Island Rail Road tracks in Kew Gardens' version of the Ponte Vecchio— that is, a bridge lined with shops. Go up the steps. At the top, you are across from the Kew Gardens Cinemas, with Art Deco lettering on the marquee, a nod to the style of the theater when it opened in the 1930s. In the neighborhood's original design, it was the location of the Kew Gardens Country Club.

● Turn right on Lefferts Blvd., traversing the "Ponte Vecchio." To withstand vibrations from the trains, the stores on Lefferts are attached through their roofs as well as on ground level. The upper connection, which has been likened to a giant curtain rod, provides the main support. At the end of the row on your right, Dani's House of Pizza has been slicing up pies topped with its trademark sweet sauce for more than half a century. A commercial hub around the rail station was laid out in the original plan for Kew Gardens.

● Turn right on Grenfell St. These next few blocks still have plenty of the lovely older homes of Kew Gardens.

● Turn left on 80th Rd.

- At Park Ln., cross and go up the steps into Forest Park. To your left is a creepily evocative statue of Job, sculpted for the 20th anniversary of Israel. Its twin is at the Holocaust memorial in Jerusalem. The Spanish Mission–style building to your right is the parks department's Queens headquarters. Known as the Overlook, it was built in 1912 when Queens finally took over administration of its own parks from Brooklyn. Novelist Henry Miller, who grew up in Brooklyn, worked in the Overlook as a parks employee in 1927 prior to his controversial literary breakthrough with *Tropic of Cancer*. Much of Forest Park's 543 acres comprise natural woodlands, but this eastern end is mostly recreational. Follow the path with the ball field on your right. When you're behind the baseball diamond, take the path to the left, go down the steps, and make a left on Park Ln. S. Don't miss the palatial houses across from the park.

- Turn right on Beverly Rd. Watch on your right for a unique mini-development: Across from #82-19, what looks like a driveway for one house is actually a cul-de-sac with a landscaped round median shared by four houses, built in the early 1920s.

- Make a right on 83rd Ave. The second house on the left stood alone atop Richmond Hill Dr., as the avenue was then named, in 1920.

- Turn right on Abingdon Rd., with a synagogue at one corner and a Jewish school at another. Kew Gardens was primarily Gentile through its first couple of decades, until European refugees began arriving in the 1930s. More recently, it is home to a growing Orthodox population, as well as Bukharian Jews from former Soviet republics in central Asia such as Uzbekistan.

- Turn left on Audley St. Right in the middle of this upscale residential block is an enormous water tower! It was erected to serve the then-new community of Richmond Hill, created by Albon Platt Man before his son Alrick developed Kew Gardens.

- Cross Metropolitan Ave. and walk on 116th St., Audley's name on the other side.

- Turn right on Grosvenor Rd., one of the neighborhood's most exclusive addresses. The mansion on your left at #115-24 is a city landmark and on the National Register of Historic Places. The African American diplomat Ralph Bunche, who was involved in establishing the United Nations, lived here for the last 30 years of his life. During that time, he was awarded the 1950 Nobel Peace Prize, becoming the first person of color so honored and the youngest recipient to date.

- Turn left on Park Ln. S. and then left on Mayfair Rd., and enjoy more of this marquee real estate. At the end of Mayfair Rd., turn around and retrace your steps. Go back on Park Ln. S. past Grosvenor Rd. to the corner of Forest Park named in honor of Raoul Wallenberg, the Swedish diplomat who saved thousands of Hungarian Jews during World War II.

- On Park Ln. S. opposite the park, get the B37 bus back to the Union Tpke. subway station. If you'd like to first cap off this walk with a nature excursion, make a left from Park Ln. S. onto Metropolitan Ave., and walk about 0.1 mile. Turn left on Forest Park Dr., and just inside the park on your right, you can follow the yellow trail through one small section of forest (the trail is about a mile long).

POINTS OF INTEREST

Dani's House of Pizza danishouseofpizza.com, 81-28 Lefferts Blvd., 718-846-2849
Forest Park Park Ln. S. and Metropolitan Ave.

route summary

1. Walk east on Queens Blvd. from the subway.
2. Turn right at Hoover Ave., which becomes 83rd Ave.
3. Turn right on Kew Gardens Rd.
4. Make a left on Mowbray Dr.
5. Cross Austin St. and walk through train-station parking lot.
6. Turn right on Lefferts Blvd.
7. Turn right on Grenfell St.
8. Make a left on 80th Rd.
9. Visit Forest Park, then go east on Park Ln. S.
10. Make a right onto Beverly Rd. and a right on 83rd Ave.
11. Make a right on Abingdon Rd.
12. Turn left on Audley St., which becomes 116th St.
13. Turn right on Grosvenor Rd.
14. Make a left on Park Ln. S.
15. Turn left on Mayfair Rd.
16. Turn around at the end, return to Park Ln. S., and go right.
17. End in Wallenberg Square, or make a left on Metropolitan Ave. to access the yellow trail in Forest Park.

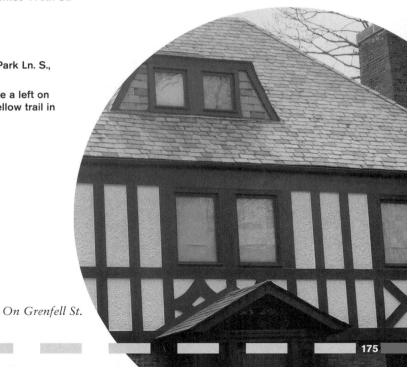

On Grenfell St.

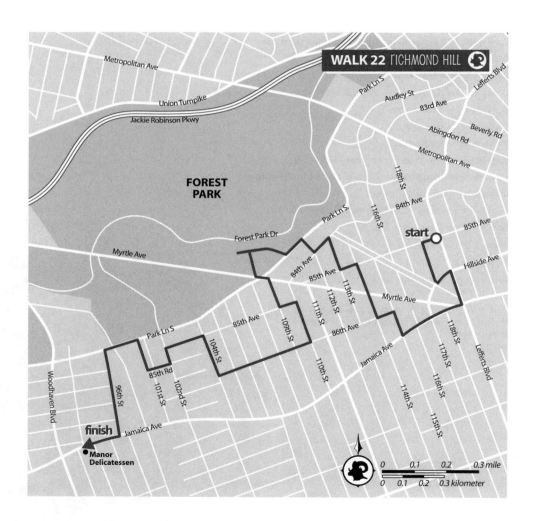

Metropolitan Ave

Park Ln S
Audley St
83rd Ave
Lefferts Blvd

Union Turnpike

Abingdon Rd
Beverly Rd

Jackie Robinson Pkwy

Metropolitan Ave

118th St

84th Ave

FOREST
PARK

85th Ave

Forest Park Dr

Park Ln S.

116th St

start

Myrtle Ave

84th Ave
85th Ave
113th St

Hillside Ave

85th Ave

112th St
111th St

Myrtle Ave

104th St
109th St

86th Ave

118th St

Park Ln S

110th St

117th St

85th Ave

Jamaica Ave

Lefferts Blvd

96th St

85th Rd
101st St
102nd St

116th St

115th St

114th St

Woodhaven Blvd

finish

Jamaica Ave

Manor
Delicatessen

0   0.1   0.2   0.3 mile

0   0.1   0.2   0.3 kilometer

22 RICHMOND HILL: a VICTORIAN VISION

BOUNDARIES: **Forest Park, Lefferts Blvd., Jamaica Ave., 95th St.**
DISTANCE: **2.9 miles**
SUBWAY: **E or F to Kew Gardens–Union Tpke., transfer to Q10 bus**

To this day, many Queens neighborhoods are described as suburbs in the city. Richmond Hill was the first to merit such a description. It was all the plan of a New York attorney named Albon Platt Man, who'd admired the hilly terrain when visiting Long Island. He bought up five farms totaling about 400 acres to create a residential community with railroad connections to Manhattan and Brooklyn, and he named the town after the London borough of Richmond upon Thames. Crusading journalist Jacob Riis, who knew a little something about how urban living could be improved, moved his family to Richmond Hill in 1886 and described it as "the most beautiful spot I had ever seen" in his memoir, *The Making of an American*. Of course, it's changed from the community Man planned: The subway's J line has supplanted the railroad for commuting; the golf course and town common are gone (so is Riis's 120th St. house). But there are some holdovers—a bevy of Victorian homes—and what a treat they are.

● Take the bus bound for JFK Airport and get out on Lefferts Blvd. at 85th Ave., next to the Church of the Resurrection. Its historical sign tells you about its milestones, in particular its connection to Jacob Riis, the Danish-born journalist who launched both the muckraking tradition and an age of urban reform with his 1890 book *How the Other Half Lives,* which he wrote while living in Richmond Hill. Theodore Roosevelt, who was NYC police commissioner when he befriended Riis, would return to the neighborhood as president of the United States in 1903, en route to Washington from the New York State Fair. In a public speech, Roosevelt told the people of Richmond Hill, "You give me strength and heart."

● Make a left on 85th Ave. Before turning on 118th St., take note of the adjacent Victorians facing you to the right. That rounded terrace on the second house is called a sleeping porch, a feature from the days before air-conditioning.

THere's even more to richmond hill

In 1895 the village of Richmond Hill absorbed the older community of Clarenceville and a hamlet called Morris Park, which had sprung up around an extravagant hotel of that name on Atlantic Ave. Almost no reminders are left of those places, save for the Morris Park name on an old park monument or two. You still might consider Richmond Hill three neighborhoods in one, though. This walk concentrates on Richmond Hill proper—the area basically coinciding with the town created by Albon Platt Man.

Farther south, around Atlantic Ave., Richmond Hill is the center of NYC's Sikh community. An estimated 15,000 Sikhs live in Richmond Hill, more than in any town or neighborhood outside India. The Sikh Cultural Society's center, encompassing a domed *gurdwara* (temple), is on 118th St. two blocks south of Atlantic Ave. In the neighborhood known as South Richmond Hill, another ethnic group predominates: Guyanese of Indian descent. Their main temple, Maha Lakshmi Mandir, is on 101st Ave. and 121st St. Every spring the Indo-Caribbean community celebrates the Hindu festival Phagwah (or Holi), spraying one another with brightly colored powdered dyes and holding a parade.

- Turn left on 118th St., passing the front of the Church of the Resurrection. At the end of the block, look through the arched rail viaduct at the marquee of the former RKO Keith's, a 2,200-seat theater that was on vaudeville's famous Orpheum circuit when it opened in 1929. The theater shut down in 1968 and is now a bingo hall.

- Turn left on Hillside Ave. Go into the library—built in 1905 on what had been the town common—to see the WPA mural *The Story of Richmond Hill,* illustrating its transition from bucolic to urbanized, with the village founders in the middle.

- Turn right on Lefferts Blvd. The landmarked Republican Club, on your left, is supposedly coming back to life as a catering hall. The clubhouse, built in 1908 with amenities like a bowling alley and archery range, hosted campaign stops by Ronald Reagan. Several presidents, including Richard Nixon and Democrat Harry S. Truman, spoke here. The building was designed by Henry Haugaard, who ran a local architecture firm with his two brothers that produced many of the Victorian homes in Richmond Hill.

- After passing beneath the Long Island Rail Road's (disused) tracks, turn right on Jamaica Ave. beneath the elevated train. An unofficial neighborhood landmark was on your right opposite 118th St.: Triangle Hofbrau, the borough's longest-running restaurant at its closing in 1999. Look for the beer-drinking gnomes carved in the doorway. Opened in 1893, it went by various names over the years. Its celebrity customers included Mae West, who lived in nearby Woodhaven, and Babe Ruth, whose favorite order was purportedly fried eel and ice cream. Triangle Hofbrau is also said to be where composer Ernest R. Ball wrote the standard "When Irish Eyes Are Smiling." On the same side, the corner building across 117th St. was meant to be seen, not obscured by an el (erected about seven years later): Ornamentation includes a figure sculpture above the 117th St. door and the building's original name high up on the avenue side.

  Across Jamaica Ave. at 116th St., look above the restaurant at the building's facade medallion, pilasters, and conical turret. It was constructed in 1900 for a bank. The bank across the street also has some detail worth noticing, particularly a pediment relief depicting a beehive (a symbol of thrift).

- Make a right on 115th St., opposite another grandiose bank. The second house on your left was the home of the Lefferts family, who sold their farmland to Albon Platt Man. Though altered, this is the original house, built sometime between 1830 and the 1860s. It was subsequently owned by Dr. William Fiske, who married Clara Riis at the Church of the Resurrection.

- Turn left on 86th Ave., the corner where Union Congregational Church has stood for more than 110 years. The congregation vacated its first church, on Hillside Ave., after only seven years because the railroad's noise and horse stables' odor proved too much of a nuisance.

- Make a right on 114th St. Toward the end of the block on your right, a house has gotten an updated exterior. If you're wondering how such a thing could have been created with the model it had right next door (at the corner), you're not alone. The next block has some classic Victorians starting halfway down on your left, and two prime specimens face each other at the end.

- Turn left on 85th Ave.

- Turn right on 113th St. The first house on the right may date as far back as 1875. Its upturned eaves, among other elements, reflect the Orientalism then in vogue in American design. This block in general offers premium Victorian viewing.

- Make a left on 84th Ave. and a right on 112th St.

- Turn left on Park Ln. S. About halfway down the block, enter Forest Park on the paved path between the metal barriers, and follow it to Memorial Dr. Just before you reach the road, watch on the right for the sign about the pine grove. Cross Memorial Dr., carefully dodging the skateboarders who love this hill, to a section where you can sit on tree trunks within a stand of pine trees.

- After communing with nature, go down Memorial Dr. to Myrtle Ave. To your right, enjoy the Zen garden, complete with stone arrangement. To your left, the statue depicting a World War I infantryman standing at a fellow soldier's grave is affectionately referred to as Buddy.

- Leaving the park, cross Park Ln. S. and Myrtle Ave. to get onto 109th St.

- Make a left on 85th Ave.

- Turn right on 110th St., with some delightful homes surrounding the intersection and continuing down the block.

- Turn right on 86th Ave., which starts with two superb houses across from each other. Another gem, at the end of the block on the right, has stained glass windows on the 109th St. side and scallop-shingled gables. If it doesn't remind you of the "painted ladies" nickname for Victorians, the bright-green home at the next corner on your right surely will. Its conical tower and circular porch link its matching street and avenue sides.

- Make a right on 104th St. Though virtually identical in profile, the two houses on your left with cute turrets present a contrast, as one goes for a barn effect with its red color and rooster weathervane.

- Turn left on 85th Ave.

- Turn left on 102nd St. The elementary school here has received landmark status from the city *and* recognition for academic excellence from the US Department of Education. It has also adopted a secondary name, the Jacqueline Kennedy Onassis School, in tribute to the former First Lady's dedication to literacy and historic preservation.

- Make a right on 85th Rd. and another right on 101st St., where a factory for the world's biggest maker of pipes and smoking supplies has been converted to residences. The 1895 complex boasts sawtooth patterning in the brickwork and a handsome central tower.

- Turn left on Park Ln. S., entering Woodhaven as you cross 98th St. The train tracks you walked under are part of the 3.5-mile segment of an abandoned LIRR route that some people are hoping to turn into an elevated park (called QueensWay), akin to Manhattan's High Line.

- Make a left on 96th St. A fine version of a rural English Gothic church was built south of 85th Rd. by St. Matthew's Episcopal, though a more historic property, the Wyckoff-Snediker Cemetery, lies behind it. The land for this town burial ground came from the adjoining farms of the Wyckoffs and the Snedikers. Construction almost swallowed it up in the 20th century, but eventually the church bought it to protect it. More recently, the church itself needed salvation, as the St. Matthew's congregation disbanded in 2011 after 110 years. Moving over from Richmond Hill, All Saints Episcopal took over the vacant church two years later.

- South of the church, turn right onto Jamaica Ave. There's an entrance to the J and Z train at 95th St., but you may want to first pick up some food at the Manor Delicatessen, between 95th and 94th Sts. Whether you want classic deli fare like a roast beef sandwich with potato salad (two of their best-sellers) or German specialties like sauerbraten, hunter's chicken, and potato pancakes, you won't find it much fresher or tastier than at this deli that's been around since 1920, when the area was heavily German.

POINTS OF INTEREST

Forest Park Myrtle Ave. and Park Ln. S.

Manor Delicatessen manordeli.com, 94-12 Jamaica Ave., 718-849-2836

route summary

1. From Lefferts Blvd., walk west on 85th Ave.
2. Turn left on 118th St.
3. Turn left on Hillside Ave.
4. Make a right on Lefferts Blvd.
5. Turn right on Jamaica Ave.
6. Turn right on 115th St.
7. Make a left on 86th Ave.
8. Turn right on 114th St.
9. Make a left on 85th Ave.
10. Turn right on 113th St.
11. Go left on 84th Ave.
12. Make a right on 112th St.
13. Go left on Park Ln. S. and into Forest Park.
14. Walk south on 109th St. from the park.
15. Make a left on 85th Ave.
16. Turn right on 110th St.
17. Make a right on 86th Ave.
18. Turn right on 104th St.
19. Turn left on 85th Ave.
20. Turn left on 102nd St.
21. Turn right on 85th Rd.
22. Make a right on 101st St.
23. Make a left on Park Ln. S.
24. Turn left on 96th St.
25. Go right on Jamaica Ave. to the train.

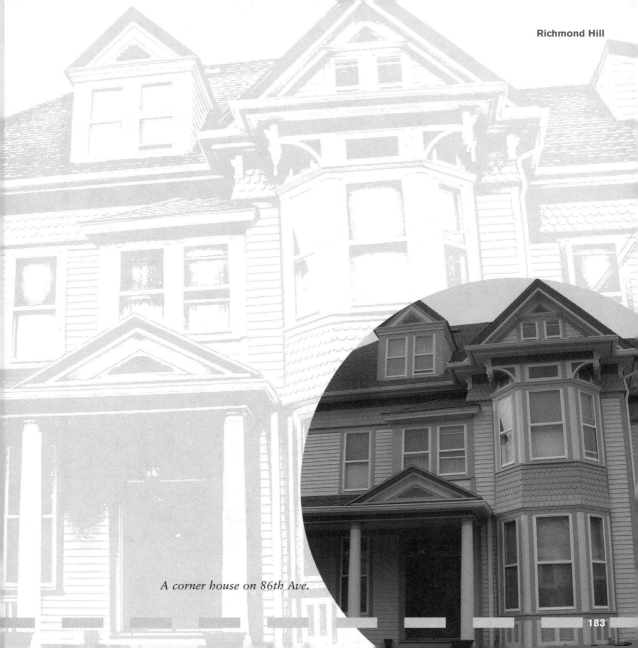

A corner house on 86th Ave.

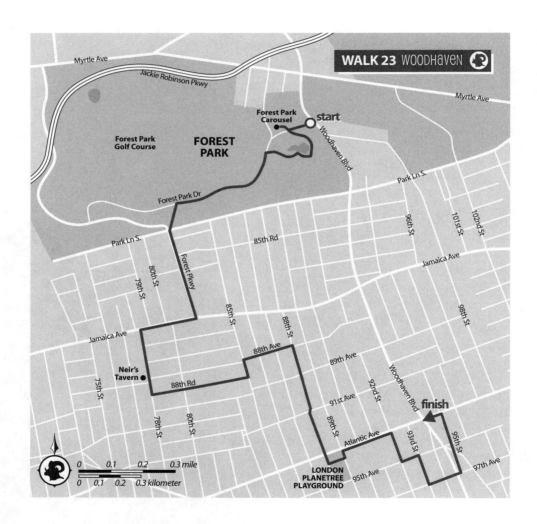

WALK 23 WOODHAVEN

Myrtle Ave
Jackie Robinson Pkwy
Myrtle Ave

Forest Park Carousel
start

Forest Park Golf Course

FOREST PARK

Park Ln S.

Forest Park Dr

Woodhaven Blvd

96th St
101st St
102nd St

Park Ln S.

85th Rd

Jamaica Ave

80th St
79th St
Forest Pkwy

98th St

85th St

88th St

Jamaica Ave

88th Ave

89th Ave

Neir's Tavern

88th Rd

91st Ave

92nd St

Woodhaven Blvd

finish

75th St

89th St

78th St
80th St

Atlantic Ave

93rd St

95th St

97th Ave

95th Ave

LONDON PLANETREE PLAYGROUND

0   0.1   0.2   0.3 mile
0   0.1   0.2   0.3 kilometer

23 WOODHAVEN: FROM FOREST PARK TO WHERE A FACTORY LEFT ITS MARK

BOUNDARIES: Forest Park, 95th St., 97th Ave., 78th St.
DISTANCE: 3 miles
SUBWAY: R or M to Woodhaven Blvd., transfer to Q11 or Q21 bus

Woodhaven borders Forest Park, and your walk starts at the park's 110-year-old wooden carousel by Daniel C. Muller, the "Michelangelo of carousel animals." The tour ends near another Woodhaven icon: the Atlantic Ave. clock tower, which managed to survive the destruction of the Lalance & Grosjean Manufacturing complex after a failed 1980s attempt to have it landmarked. Without Lalance & Grosjean, many would tell you, there would be no Woodhaven. The kitchenware maker set up shop in quiet, sparsely populated Woodhaven in 1863 with fewer than a hundred employees, and by the turn of the century employed about 2,000 people and had given rise to a factory town. Woodhaven originated, however, with the 1830s plan of Connecticut businessman John Pitkin to create an independent city, named East New York, spanning the Brooklyn–Queens border south of Cypress Hills. He had to abandon the whole project because of the economic Panic of 1837, and East New York ended up as a neighborhood of Brooklyn. The eastern section Pitkin had laid out became Woodhaven.

- Get off the bus at Forest Park Dr. and go into the park next to the bus stop. Ahead on your right is a path to the carousel, which has won landmark designation from the city. It's one of only two intact carousels by Muller, who was renowned for anatomical detail and realistic rather than fanciful outfitting of the horses. Each animal is estimated to be worth at least $150,000; most of Muller's carousels were dismantled and sold off in parts (Ohio's Cedar Point amusement park has the other complete one). The carousel includes a German-made calliope organ, paintings of Queens scenes of yesteryear, and carved angels above the mirrors at its center. From its north side, you can see the greenhouse, where plants for all of the borough's parks are grown.

- Return to Forest Park Dr. and make a left. Close to the park entrance, on your right you'll find the path around PFC Laurence Strack Memorial Pond. The entrance sign tells you the history of the site, from the pond's formation by receding glaciers to the ill-fated original memorial to Private Strack. Follow the path downhill and walk with the low log barrier on your right. The path slopes farther downhill and brings you to boulders bordering a "beach." This is not the only kettle pond in Queens that was landfilled for one reason or another only to be later restored; it's now home to turtles, frogs, and such birds as hawks and herons. Take the asphalt path from the patio overlooking the pond, and proceed to Forest Park Dr.

- With the parking lot in front of you, make a left. On your right is a 1920 band shell. Forest Park's music tradition was started by George Seuffert Sr., a German-born violinist (and friend of John Philip Sousa) who organized a military band that gave concerts here before the band shell, now named for him, was even erected.

- Continue past the band shell about 0.25 mile on Forest Park Dr., designed by Frederick Law Olmsted of Central Park fame. To your right as you walk, beyond the chain-link fence, is the 18-hole Forest Park Golf Course. When you reach stairs on your left, go down them through the woods and all the way to Park Ln. S.

- Cross Park Ln. S. and begin walking on Forest Pkwy., which was created as an upscale residential development of that name in 1900. Its boulevard width was one of the deluxe amenities it offered; another was pavement at a time when dirt roads were the norm.

- On the left at 85th Dr. is the local library, dating to 1924. It was the last of seven libraries built in Queens through an endowment from steel magnate Andrew Carnegie, who donated more than $5 million to New York City in 1901 for the construction of 65 libraries. Queens, with its small population compared with Manhattan and Brooklyn in that pre–Queensboro Bridge era, got less than 5% of the funds. Woodhaven also has one of three Queens post offices with WPA art—if it's open, go inside to see the *First Amendment* mural. Opposite the post office at 86th Rd., in front of the bank is Woodhaven's version of a town square, centered on a World War II honor-roll monument. Look across the street to the top of the corner building (also a bank) where FOREST PARKWAY is engraved in the cornice.

- Turn right on Jamaica Ave., which has some august old buildings, though they can get obscured by signs, their proximity to the el, and the general hubbub of this commercial thoroughfare. Look above the discount-store awning at #80-30, for example, for the inscription THE LEADER-OBSERVER, the name of the local newspaper for whom the building was constructed circa 1914. The store at #80-16 gets its broad, high building from the Haven, where generations of Woodhavenites grew up seeing movies.

- Turn left onto 78th St. At Neir's Tavern, on your right at 88th Ave., you can have a sand-wich named after a movie shot on-site: Several scenes in the Mob classic *Goodfellas* featuring Robert De Niro were filmed in the bar, and Ben Stiller meets with Téa Leoni here in *Tower Heist.* But Neir's biggest claim to fame is as the oldest bar in Queens. Nobody's quite sure when the tavern first opened—in the 1850s or 1830s, possibly as early as 1829—but it's had several names; the current one honors its owners from 1898 to 1967, who also operated a bowling alley, ballroom, and lodging in the building. Mae West, who lived nearby on 88th St., performed at Neir's before she became a movie star, and the current bar is full of West memorabilia. The latest owners have resumed the live-entertainment tradition and restored its interior decor. Beers are drawn from a 100-plus-year-old tap system whose coils sit in ice, because it's from the days before electricity. The logo, meanwhile, pays homage to the bar's earliest years, when it thrived on the patronage of horse-racing fans. One of the country's premier racetracks, Union Course, was across the street from 1821 until the 1870s. Union Course is depicted in Currier and Ives prints, and its customers kept three hotels on Jamaica Ave. in busi-ness. Its races often pitted horses from the North and South against each other. After Union Course was demolished, real estate developers promptly snatched up its former grounds, and by 1910 they'd filled the area with houses.

- Turn left on 88th Rd. At 80th St., a white picket fence surrounds a nice house on your right that has some intricate woodworking on its wraparound porch.

- Make a left on 85th St., then a right on 88th Ave. St. Thomas the Apostle Church casts a presence on the blocks branching off from its 87th St. corner, due to both its imposing structure and its numerous related buildings, including a school and con-vent. It also converted a former movie theater on Jamaica Ave. to a social hall, which has been used to handle overflow attendance at Mass.

- Make a right on 88th St., where you'll see that Tudor half-timbering is not limited to the ritzier neighborhoods of Queens.

- Cross Atlantic Ave. and go to the left. Turn right on 89th St. and enter London Plan-etree Playground. Enjoy watching the daredevils in the $1.8 million skate park that was constructed in mid-2013. Afterward, return to Atlantic Ave. and go to your right. The brick building on your right at 90th St. is a remnant of Lalance & Grosjean's main building, which fronted Atlantic all the way to the clock tower. Originally Manhattan-based importers, Lalance & Grosjean became the first American manufacturer of agate ware (enameled utensils made of metal) and maintained operations in Woodhaven until they went out of business in the 1950s. The company refined the process of stamping—in which a piece would be made from a single sheet of metal—and was supplied by its own steel mill in Pennsylvania. It also made products of tin, copper, brass, and iron, including wartime military supplies. At one time there was an aerial bridge from the second and third stories of the clock tower to the building across 92nd St. Products were enameled and finished in that building, which now houses a Burger King and grocery store. Its 1899 construction made Lalance & Grosjean the world's largest stamping works.

● Turn right at the clock tower and walk through the parking lot. There is one other building here: a single story high, with a half-dozen storefronts. A series of elongated brick "sheds" like this used to be part of the factory, and all this parking space was occupied by a multistory building three blocks long.

● Turn left on 95th Ave. as you leave the shopping center. The old buildings in this vicinity date to the 19th century, when a village sprang up around the factory. The crown jewel of the old Woodhaven village survivors is the Wyckoff at 93rd St., a Queen Anne–Romanesque mash-up erected in 1889 for a bank and real estate company.

● Make a right on 93rd St. The second freestanding house on your right was constructed in the 1850s—at least the south section was; the main part with a porch was added later.

● Turn left on 97th Ave. Cross Woodhaven Blvd.

● Make a left on Woodhaven Blvd. Past some nondescript residences stands an elegantly old-fashioned house with a dormered turret. It looks out of place in its present-day surroundings but was typical in the late 19th century, when there were several mansions off the boulevard. The best view of this house is from the tip of its triangular plot, where Woodhaven Blvd. and 95th St. meet.

● Continue north on 95th St., where another attractive old house (with a flagpole on its lawn) stands on the other side of the traffic island.

● **Turn left on Atlantic Ave. and go back to Woodhaven Blvd. for a bus. Take any bus northbound for the J, R, or M train, southbound for the A.**

POINTS OF INTEREST

Forest Park Carousel forestparkcarousel.com, Woodhaven Blvd. and Forest Park Dr.
Neir's Tavern neirstavern.com, 87-48 78th St., 718-296-0600
London Planetree Playground Atlantic Ave. and 88th St.

ROUTE SUMMARY

1. Enter Forest Park at the Woodhaven gate.
2. After walking around the carousel and pond, walk west on Forest Park Dr.
3. Go left through the woods to Park Ln. S.
4. Walk south on Forest Pkwy.
5. Make a right on Jamaica Ave.
6. Turn left on 78th St.
7. Turn left on 88th Rd.
8. Make a left on 85th St.
9. Turn right on 88th Ave.
10. Make a right on 88th St.
11. Go left on Atlantic Ave.
12. Enter London Planetree Playground at 89th St. and Atlantic Ave., and exit at the same place.
14. Head east on Atlantic Ave.
15. Make a right on 92nd St.
16. Turn left on 95th Ave.
17. Turn right on 93rd St.
18. Make a left on 97th Ave.
19. Cross Woodhaven Blvd. and go left.
20. Merge onto 95th St.
21. Go left on Atlantic Ave. to Woodhaven Blvd.

The Wyckoff, built in 1889

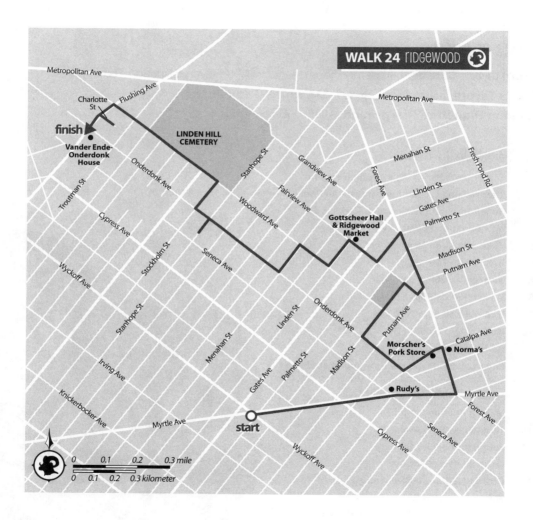

WALK 24 ridgewood

Metropolitan Ave

Charlotte St

Flushing Ave

finish

Vander Ende-
Onderdonk
House

LINDEN HILL
CEMETERY

Metropolitan Ave

Stanhope St

Grandview Ave

Menahan St

Forest Ave

Linden St

Gates Ave

Palmetto St

Fresh Pond Rd

Troutman St

Onderdonk Ave

Fairview Ave

Woodward Ave

Madison St

Putnam Ave

Cypress Ave

Seneca Ave

Gottscheer Hall
& Ridgewood
Market

Wyckoff Ave

Stockholm St

Stanhope St

Putnam Ave

Menahan St

Linden St

Onderdonk Ave

Catalpa Ave

Irving Ave

Putnam Ave

Morscher's
Pork Store

Norma's

Gates Ave

Palmetto St

Madison St

Myrtle Ave

Knickerbocker Ave

Rudy's

Forest Ave

start

Myrtle Ave

Wyckoff Ave

Cypress Ave

Seneca Ave

0   0.1   0.2   0.3 mile
0   0.1   0.2   0.3 kilometer

24 RIDGEWOOD: FOLLOW THE YELLOW-BRICK ABODES

BOUNDARIES: **Flushing Ave., Forest Ave., Myrtle Ave., Wyckoff Ave.**
DISTANCE: **3 miles**
SUBWAY: **L or M to Myrtle–Wyckoff Aves.**

Ridgewood might be both the most historic and the most au courant place in Queens. The Greater Ridgewood Historical Society is headquartered in a house dating to the 1650s, and the National Register of Historic Places lists 18 different districts within Ridgewood. Yet you're also likely to find Ridgewood on any list of up-and-coming neighborhoods in New York City, typically under a headline like "The new Williamsburg!" Gentrification has pushed the hip and artsy across the Brooklyn border in search of affordable, low-key cool. Once upon a time Ridgewood shared a different population with neighboring Bushwick and Williamsburg: German immigrants, who began settling in the area in the 1880s and were still the majority into the 1960s. They've dropped to less than 10% of the Ridgewood population, though the German American School (established 1892) and the Steuben Society (since 1919) are both still open on Fresh Pond Rd. What really dominates Ridgewood is not a particular group of people but a group of houses: the Mathews Model Flats, yellow-brick row houses built by the hundreds (by developer Gustave X. Mathews) between 1905 and 1915.

● The subway station is in Brooklyn—the border between boroughs is at the Myrtle–Wyckoff intersection—but you begin at a Queens address, 54-00 Myrtle Ave., and walk east on Myrtle. The tallest building on your right, its roof lined with stone seashells, used to be the 2,700-seat RKO Madison theater. The small park across the avenue, Venditti Square, is named in honor of a policeman who was killed in front of the restaurant while staking out an alleged mobster.

Two blocks farther on Myrtle, the Ridgewood Theatre, on your left, was the longest-running movie house in the country when it shuttered in March 2008. It opened before movies had sound, in 1916, and was designed by Thomas Lamb, the premier architect of lavish cinemas, with 2,500 seats. At its closing, it was a grungy five-screen theater. The exterior has been landmarked, and there's talk of a residential conversion by the latest owner.

● Continue past the theater to Ridgewood's elegant World War I memorial. Service-men guided by angels and gods are portrayed in the tall bronze bas-reliefs that curve around a cylindrical monument inscribed with poignant sentiments. The drugstore across Myrtle occupies a neoclassical building erected in 1910 for Ridgewood National Bank—and I recommended seeing it from the inside. Louis Berger, the main architect of Mathews housing, was one of the bank founders.

There are a couple of good places early on this walk to satisfy a sweet tooth. You can see one from Myrtle to your left on Seneca Ave., Rudy's. It was strictly a German patisserie (a *konditorei*, as the awning says) when it opened in 1934, and you can still get strudel and *bienenstich* cake there, but inventory has expanded to eclairs, cannoli, scones, and pretty much any kind of cake or cookie or tart, plus gelato.

● Go a few more blocks on Myrtle Ave. and you'll find another neoclassical bank build-ing at another three-road intersection, where George St. and Forest Ave. meet Myrtle. It has a clock within an archway above the front door and a balustrade along the roof, like the former Ridgewood National Bank. But Ridgewood Savings Bank has weath-ered demographic shifts and bank consolidation to remain, under the same name, in these 1929 headquarters. The other date engraved on the facade, 1921, is the year that a group of German American businessmen opened the bank in a converted bar on the same site. From the wrought iron clock to the marble floors, there's all kinds of great detail to this building; don't overlook the human figures in the capitals of the window columns.

● Turn left on Forest Ave.

● At Catalpa Ave., you may want to pop into Norma's on your right for a baked treat or premium coffee. This cozy café helps promote the arts community (small artist-run galleries are scattered around the neighborhood) and sells products by local crafts-people. But head in the other direction on Catalpa, toward the large church. Watch on your left for Morscher's Pork Store, the neighborhood's last German butcher shop. Its signage includes an illustration and quote from a Brothers Grimm story in which the command "Little table, spread thyself" (that's the German phrase on the sign) prompts a table to magically set itself with a place setting and a serving of wine and meats. Morscher's makes wursts from German, Hungarian, Austrian, Slovenian,

Serbian, Italian, and Swiss recipes, and carries a huge variety of other meats and grocery products too.

This side of Catalpa also has Serbian, Islamic, and Polish businesses, but St. Matthias Church dominates the block. Standing taller than any other structure in south Ridgewood, the majestic copper-roofed church is surmounted with a wedding-cake arrangement that entails columns, clocks, pediments, and a small dome. Pope John Paul II, depicted in a statue in the churchyard, was a national hero to the large Polish membership of St. Matthias.

● Turn right on Onderdonk Ave. This street and the ones that cross it are full of Mathews Model Flats. Their archetypal exterior features two colors of brick, round-arched windows on the third floor, and decoratively carved doorway molding. They were called model flats because they provided a higher standard of living for the working class than otherwise available at the time. Mathews's buildings typically had two apartments per floor, and every room had at least one window. They were such an improvement in tenement housing that they were exhibited at the 1915 world's fair in San Francisco.

● Make a right on Madison St. All this yellow brick was made by B. Kreischer & Sons of Staten Island, from clay mined in the same area where the brick factory was located. After crossing Woodward Ave., look on the ground to your right for remnants of trolley tracks, which follow the same path as the M train overhead. The trolleys ceased operating in the 1940s.

● Turn right on Fairview Ave., then left on Putnam Ave.

On Myrtle Ave.

- Make a left on Forest Ave. The Romanian Orthodox church on your right occupies a 1906 mansion that was once the most impressive residence in town. Note the keystone busts on the top windows. On the next block, the single wood-frame house at #66-45 is from 1885, prior to the mass development of brick row houses in the neighborhood. At the next corner, Forest Pork Store continues to make German-style sausages and smoked meats here in Ridgewood—but for the wholesale trade (the retail shop closed in 2007). From Società Concordia Partanna, a Sicilian social club, at #66-23, you have a good vantage on the angled facades across Forest Ave.

- Make a left on Palmetto St.

- Turn right on Fairview Ave. Across Gates Ave. on your right, Gottscheer Hall could be described as a saloon or a community center or a catering hall, but none of those—while accurate—captures its importance in the lives of a good portion of the Ridgewood population for the past 90 years. Many of the Germans who've resided in Ridgewood came from Gottschee, a region of present-day Slovenia that used to be part of the Austrian Empire. From this building, they organized fundraising and advocacy campaigns on behalf of Gottscheers still in Europe who were displaced by World War II, and provided support and assistance to their compatriots living in the area. Gottscheer Hall's bar and grill are open to the public, and many non-Gottscheer groups have held events in the ballroom. It's also the home of the new Ridgewood Market, a monthly showcase for local artists, chefs, and antiques dealers.

- Turn left on Linden St. Architect Louis Berger is responsible for thousands of the Mathews houses in Ridgewood, but only a few of them have faces sculpted above the second- and third-floor windows, as on this block.

- Make a right on Woodward Ave. St. Mary & St. Antonios, on your left at Grove St., was the third Coptic Orthodox church in the United States when it was established in the 1970s; there are now more than 200 of these Egyptian Christian churches. St. Mary & St. Antonios expanded to a second house of worship—a century-old church a half mile away—in 2011, the year the congregation doubled in size due to mass emigration of Egyptians in the wake of the Arab Spring revolution.

- Go left on Menahan St. About a third of the way down the block on your left, the Romanian American organization Banatul has adapted a turn-of-the-century taproom for its clubhouse.

- Turn right on Onderdonk Ave. You should see the 165-foot twin towers of St. Aloysius Catholic Church looming ahead of you—and the Empire State Building in the distance.

- Go left on Stanhope St. to St. Aloysius's convent next to the parking lot. It was built in 1893, shortly after the parish was founded.

- Return to Onderdonk Ave. and proceed to the front of the church. Try to get a look at its interior, even if only through the glass doors in the lobby. This building, made of Kreischer brick, was begun in 1907 and, not surprisingly given its size and detail, took nearly a decade to complete. Today St. Aloysius conducts Mass in English, Polish, and Spanish.

- Make a right on Stockholm St., observing the change in pavement. These are not the cobblestone paving blocks you find in other old NYC neighborhoods; they are Kreischer bricks, which makes this a yellow-brick road—with landmark protection no less. The landmark designation report recognized its "intact, harmonious, and architecturally distinguished . . . working-class dwellings," namely the two-story bowfront houses, which were designed by Louis Berger, as were the apartment buildings at each corner with Woodward Ave.

- Turn left on Woodward Ave. and walk alongside Linden Hill Cemetery. If you look in, you'll see graves in English, Spanish, Italian, German, Chinese, French, Polish, and Hungarian. While the city-designated historic district covers only Stockholm St., the national historic district includes DeKalb Ave. and Hart St. to your left. Both have fairly uniform groups of houses. The west side of Hart, facing you, offers something different: recessed entrances and decorative gables. As you continue on Woodward, more of the Manhattan skyline comes into view.

- Turn left on Flushing Ave. It ain't pretty, so for a respite from the barbed wire and truck noise, go down Charlotte St. on your left. Surprise! It's a cul-de-sac of cute curved-bay brick row houses—developed when Flushing Ave. was still mostly residential. Until almost the middle of the 20th century, several old farmsteads remained along this part of the avenue.

- Go back to Flushing Ave. and continue in the direction you were headed. The sole surviving Dutch Colonial farmhouse, the Vander Ende–Onderdonk House, sits within a spacious yard at the next corner. The shingle-roofed fieldstone house was constructed in 1709 on the foundations of a wooden house that had been erected around 1650. Now open for tours and special events under the aegis of the Greater Ridgewood Historical Society, the house contains furnished rooms, a "general store" display of period objects, and an exhibit of archeological finds from the property. On the grounds are a vegetable garden, chicken coop, picnic grove, and Arbitration Rock, perhaps the same boulder that was placed in the road in the 1700s to demarcate the border between Brooklyn and Queens.

● Across Flushing Ave. from the Onderdonk House, take the B57 bus for connection to the L, M, or J train (stay on the bus longer, and you can connect to practically every subway line in Downtown Brooklyn).

POINTS OF INTEREST

Rudy's rudysbakeryandcafe.com, 905 Seneca Ave., 718-821-5890

Norma's cafenormas.com, 59-02 Catalpa Ave., 347-294-0185

Morscher's Pork Store morschersporkstore.com, 58-44 Catalpa Ave., 718-821-1040

Gottscheer Hall gottscheerhall.com, 657 Fairview Ave., 718-366-3030

Ridgewood Market ridgewoodmarket.com, 657 Fairview Ave., 347-460-7549

Vander Ende–Onderdonk House onderdonkhouse.org, 1820 Flushing Ave., 718-456-1776

route summary

1. Walk east on Myrtle Ave. from Wyckoff Ave.
2. Go left on Forest Ave.
3. Turn left on Catalpa Ave.
4. Turn right on Onderdonk Ave.
5. Turn right on Madison St.
6. Make a right on Fairview Ave.
7. Turn left on Putnam Ave.
8. Make a left on Forest Ave.
9. Make a left on Palmetto St.
10. Make a right on Fairview Ave.
11. Turn left on Linden St.
12. Make a right on Woodward Ave.
13. Turn left on Menahan St.
14. Make a right on Onderdonk Ave.
15. Go left on Stanhope St., then turn around.
16. Turn left on Onderdonk Ave.
17. Make a right on Stockholm St.
18. Make a left on Woodward Ave.
19. Go left on Flushing Ave., dipping in and out of Charlotte St. en route to the Onderdonk House.

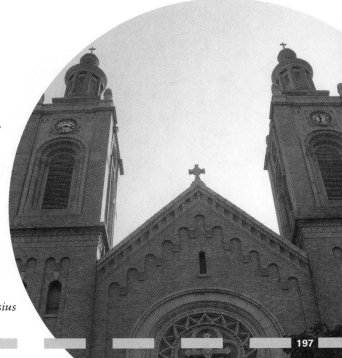

The towers of St. Aloysius

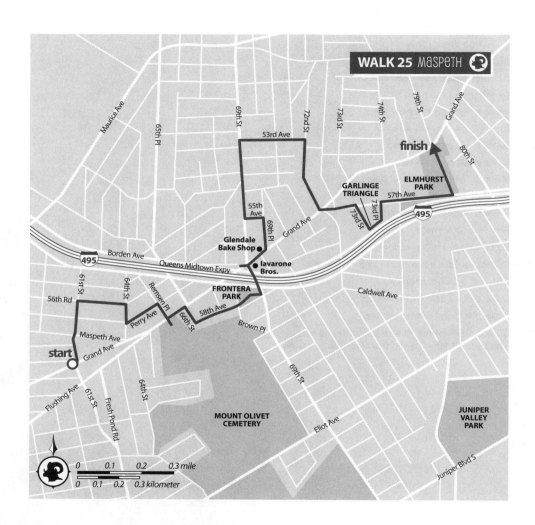

WALK 25 MASPETH

finish

ELMHURST
PARK

GARLINGE
TRIANGLE

57th Ave

53rd Ave

69th St

72nd St

73rd St

74th St

79th St

80th St

Grand Ave

73rd Pl

73rd St

55th
Ave

69th Pl

Grand Ave

Glendale
Bake Shop

Iavarone
Bros.

FRONTERA
PARK

Maurice Ave

65th Pl

Borden Ave

495

Queens Midtown Expy

495

Caldwell Ave

61st St

64th St

Remsen Pl

Perry Ave

66th St

58th Ave

Brown Pl

56th Rd

Maspeth Ave

start

Grand Ave

Flushing Ave

61st St

Fresh Pond Rd

64th St

69th St

Eliot Ave

MOUNT OLIVET
CEMETERY

JUNIPER
VALLEY
PARK

Juniper Blvd S

0   0.1   0.2   0.3 mile

0   0.1   0.2   0.3 kilometer

25 MaSPeTH: SMaLL-TOWN PriDe

BOUNDARIES: 53rd Ave., Elmhurst Park, 58th Ave., 61st St.
DISTANCE: 2.5 miles
SUBWAY: L to Grand St. (Brooklyn), transfer to Rego Park–bound Q59 bus

So close yet so far—that's how Maspeth seems. It borders Brooklyn and is the second neighborhood in coming from Manhattan. But no subway goes there, and the neighborhood is hemmed in by cemeteries and industrial districts that can be desolate in off-hours. Outside the truck-route-and-warehouse territory, a small-town ambience prevails in much of residential Maspeth. Its aesthetic lapses notwithstanding, Maspeth has proved invaluable to New York City. The first land deed ever issued on Long Island, in 1642, covered the Maspeth area (it got its name from an American Indian tribe called Mespat or Mespachtes). DeWitt Clinton, arguably the most important statesman New York has produced, resided in Maspeth while serving as NYC mayor. Innumerable goods and services that New Yorkers rely on every day are stored, handled, or prepared in Maspeth. For generations it's been a place where immigrants gain a foothold in America. And what about Maspeth's sacrifice on September 11, 2001? Nineteen firefighters from Maspeth's Squad 288/Hazmat Company 1 gave their lives, the biggest loss of any firehouse in the city.

● From the subway station in Williamsburg, the bus twice crosses Newtown Creek, which forms a natural, albeit toxic, boundary between Queens and Brooklyn. (In the late 1970s, decades after the creek's heyday as an industrial channel, a massive underground oil spill was discovered—upward of 17 million gallons, which they've been pumping out since 1995.) A 1903 steel-truss swing bridge brings you into Queens. Get off the bus on Grand Ave. at 61st St.

● Make a left onto 61st. The neighborhood's Polish flavor becomes evident within one block, as you approach St. Stanislaus Kostka Church, positioned diagonally at the right corner with Maspeth Ave. St. Stans, as everyone calls it, is the oldest Catholic congregation in Maspeth, established in 1872 and named for a Polish saint. Its membership has diversified in recent decades, and it now holds a weekly Spanish-language Mass. Continuing on 61st St., you pass Polish shops at the next two corners.

- Turn right on 56th Rd. Holy Cross Church was founded by Polish immigrants, who chipped in to cover construction costs for this 1913 California-mission-meets-fairy-tale structure. Parishioners were thrilled when Karol Wojtyla, the archbishop of Krakow, visited in 1969, and even more thrilled when he became Pope John Paul II a decade later. The pope was sculpted at his friendliest for the statue in front of the rectory. Near the end of the block, look up at the bilingual inscription on the building on your right identifying it (in Polish) as the Polish National Home, a cultural and community center.

- Go right on 64th St. and then left onto Perry Ave. for the unique-looking Transfiguration Church. Both Modernistic and Lithuanian-inflected, the glass-front A-frame has a wavy roof above the entryway. The words at the doors are Lithuanian for "my house is a house of prayer." In addition to folk art inside the church, a wayside shrine stands on the lawn of the church house to the right. These wooden totems are placed in roads, farms, fields, and forests around Lithuania as memorials or commemorations of joyous events. For instance, this wayside, dedicated to those who lost their lives, depicts birds (which symbolize reincarnation) and the Pietà (the Virgin Mary mourning over the dead body of Christ), as well as the so-called Sorrowful or Pensive Christ, a common icon on Lithuanian woodcarvings.

- Turn right on Remsen Pl., and go straight across Grand Ave. into Mount Olivet Cemetery to see its 1870s stone gatehouse. In the 19th century, before public parks were developed on a large scale, people would come to garden cemeteries for the greenery and open air. Mount Olivet has winding drives, abundant horticulture, and one of the highest points in Queens. The cemetery contains a special lot for Civil War veterans and their wives.

- Go back to Grand Ave. Across from the cemetery entrance, the building with the florist at street level dates to 1851, when it opened as an inn for Long Island farmers on their way to and from market in Brooklyn.

- Make a right on Grand Ave. and another right on 66th St.

- Turn left on 58th Ave., where you find some well-kept turn-of-the century houses—some of them with fine porch woodworking. The block's trophy property is the corner house on your left at Brown Pl., built in the 1880s.

- Cross Brown Pl. and enter Frontera Park, refurbished with a firefighting theme a year after Maspeth's huge loss on 9/11. Walk past the basketball courts and flagpole to the children's play area replicating an antique fire engine pulled by horses. Look amid the play equipment for the pretend storefronts of a bank and a barbershop. Longtime resident Frank Frontera, the park's namesake, was a barber who cofounded Maspeth Federal Savings and served as a volunteer fireman until his death at age 91.

- Continue through the park to 69th St., and cross the street to the smaller park. Look for more horse imagery on the fence posts flanking the path: an homage to public transit of the 19th century, the horsecar. A popular route through Maspeth took people to Calvary Cemetery; in the Brooklyn-bound direction, riders from Queens would pile on in the summer to connect to the railroad out to Coney Island.

- Follow 69th St. across the Queens Midtown Expy. (western spur of the Long Island Expy.) and then across Borden Ave. to the plaza in front of Maspeth Federal Savings. Its centerpiece is a tripartite monument honoring the Squad 288/Hazmat 1 firefighters and the six Maspeth residents who died on 9/11, with artifacts from Ground Zero on display. Facing the memorial, you can look directly at the World Trade Center. If you'd like to pay respects at the 100-year-old firehouse itself, it's just around the corner on 68th St. if you follow Borden Ave. behind the monuments.

- Take Grand Ave. north from the memorial plaza. Immediately on your right at 69th St., the Italian grocery lavarone Bros. prepares plenty of ready-to-eat foods, such as heroes, hot entrées, and deli fare. On the other

Mural at Borden Ave. and Grand Ave.

side of the avenue at #63-25, neighborhood classic Glendale Bake Shop has a large selection of cookies, cakes, turnovers, and the like, but its No. 1 item is the pretzel roll.

- Turn left on 69th Pl. On your right, the second house after the garages is a nice 1911 model with roomy porch and keystone upper window. The attached brick houses a few doors down were constructed in the 1920s as a Tudor ensemble.

- Turn left on 55th Ave., beside a beautifully crafted and maintained Tudor. This short block has at least four different types of residences, including a couple of Brooklyn-style row houses with stoops and ornamented cornices.

- Turn right on 69th St. On the right, parapets and matching doorway and gable roofs dress up the tract houses. Farther north, the mansard roof at 53rd Dr. dates the building as older than many of its neighbors. In some places, variety exists within one property, like on your right past 53rd Rd., where houses that are brick at the bottom have a shingled top floor.

- Make a right on 53rd Ave.

- Turn right on 72nd St. Maspeth Town Hall, on your left, never functioned as such, and the date on its sign is inaccurate too. It was built as a school in 1897 and went through several other identities, as well as periods of neglect, ultimately to be resurrected as a community center.

- Make a left onto Grand Ave. At the sidewalk clock, walk through Garlinge Triangle past its World War I memorial and onto 57th Ave.

- Turn right on 73rd St. A curiosity can be found at 57th Rd.: the Quick Brown Fox Triangle. Yes, it's named for that famous sentence that contains every letter of the alphabet, "The quick brown fox jumps over the lazy dog." But does the area have some connection to typesetters? Nah. It was just a former parks commissioner having some fun: He added whimsical place-names around the city. Officially within the Long Island Expy., this park (complete with fox statue) has to be one of the most bizarre choices for an outdoor respite.

- Walk east on the Queens Midtown Expy. (the opposite direction as the traffic), and turn left on 73rd Pl.

- Turn right on 57th Ave. You move from Maspeth into Elmhurst as you cross the railroad overpass. Elmhurst Park is your final destination. This lovely 6-acre greensward was developed on the most famous site in Elmhurst, a place familiar to people who never even set foot in the neighborhood: the Elmhurst gas tanks. Two enormous 275-foot-wide cylinders, the tanks were visible from the Long Island Expy. Between that and their location just a few miles out of the Manhattan tunnel, they made a convenient reference point for traffic reports; "backed up at the tanks" was a common refrain on the radio for years. Natural gas isn't stored in huge tanks anymore, but in smaller pressurized containers, and in the 1990s, the gas company dismantled them and sold the land to the city for $1. It took $20 million, land decontamination, and the planting of some 600 trees to turn it into a park. The design is both environmental and clever: Children's play equipment is shaped like models of atoms, in keeping with the energy theme; the comfort station's shape recalls the gas tanks.

- After enjoying the park, exit at its other (north) end, Grand Ave. At the bus stop just outside the park, take the Q58 and Q59 to the R and M. If you want to return to the L and M station where you started, take the Q59 in the other direction.

POINTS OF INTEREST

Frontera Park Brown Pl. and 58th Ave.

Iavarone Bros. ibfoods.com, 69-00 Grand Ave., 718-639-3623

Glendale Bake Shop 69-25 Grand Ave., 718-457-2006

Elmhurst Park Grand Ave. and 79th St.

route summary

1. Walk north on 61st St. from Grand Ave.

2. Make a right on 56th Rd.

3. Turn right on 64th St.

4. Turn left on Perry Ave.

5. Make a right on Remsen Pl. Cross Grand Ave. to see Mount Olivet Cemetery, and return to Grand Ave.

6. Make a right on Grand Ave.

7. Go right at 66th St.

8. Turn left on 58th Ave.

9. Enter Frontera Park at Brown Pl.

10. Exit the park on 69th St., and go left.

11. Head north on Grand Ave. from 69th St.

12. Turn left on 69th Pl.

13. Make a left on 55th Ave.

14. Turn right on 69th St.

15. Turn right on 53rd Ave.

16. Turn right on 72nd St.

17. Make a left on Grand Ave.

18. Go through Garlinge Triangle onto 57th Ave.

19. Turn right on 73rd St.

20. Turn left on Queens Midtown Expy. service road.

21. Turn left on 73rd Pl.

22. Make a right on 57th Ave.

23. Walk through Elmhurst Park to Grand Ave.

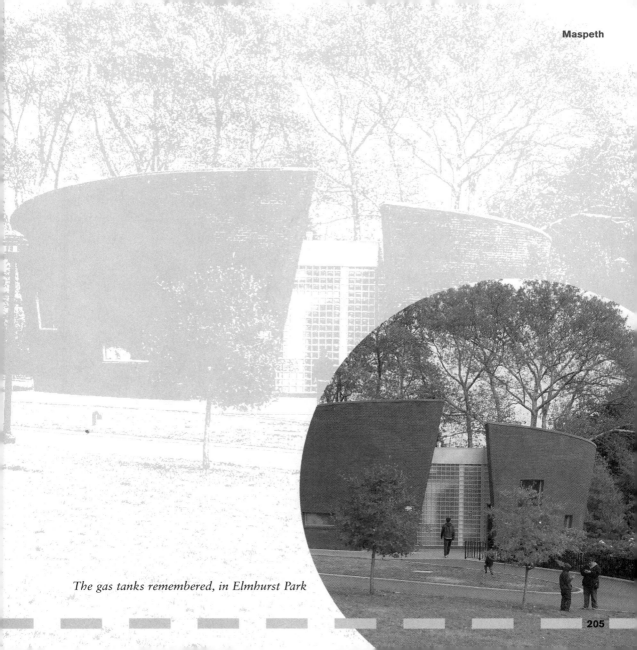

The gas tanks remembered, in Elmhurst Park

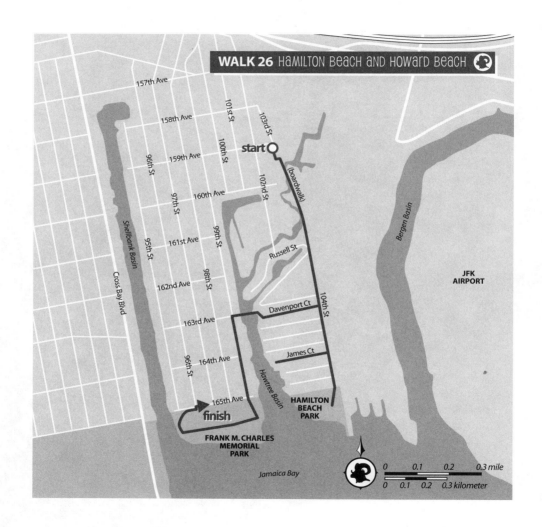

WALK 26 HAMILTON BEACH AND HOWARD BEACH

157th Ave

158th Ave

159th Ave

160th Ave

161st Ave

162nd Ave

163rd Ave

164th Ave

165th Ave

101st St

100th St

102nd St

103rd St

96th St

97th St

99th St

98th St

96th St

95th St

Shellbank Basin

Cross Bay Blvd

start

(boardwalk)

Russell St

Davenport Ct

James Ct

104th St

Hawtree Basin

HAMILTON BEACH PARK

finish

FRANK M. CHARLES MEMORIAL PARK

Jamaica Bay

Bergen Basin

JFK AIRPORT

0   0.1   0.2   0.3 mile
0   0.1   0.2   0.3 kilometer

26 HAMILTON BEACH AND HOWARD BEACH: TUCKED AWAY IN JAMAICA BAY

BOUNDARIES: 159th Ave., 104th St., Jamaica Bay, 95th St.
DISTANCE: 2.4 miles
SUBWAY: A to Howard Beach–JFK Airport

When Hamilton Beach made the news as one of the places hard-hit by Superstorm Sandy in 2012, it was the first time that many people had heard of the neighborhood. Hamilton Beach lies amid basins and channels of Jamaica Bay, abutting train tracks and John F. Kennedy International Airport. Despite its proximity to all those comings and goings, Hamilton Beach has been relatively untouched by the outside world, i.e., urbanization. Pictures in a 1908 newspaper profile of this "quaint creekside settlement" show scenes that don't look that much different today. Eventually it became part of Howard Beach, and today many nonresidents are unfamiliar with the distinctions among communities within Howard Beach. This walk visits the two east of Cross Bay Blvd., Hamilton Beach and so-called Old Howard Beach. It's a route designed primarily to take you into far-off corners of New York City and showcase a lesser-trod stretch of NYC's waterfront.

- Your first inkling that Hamilton Beach is different from other places in New York City is its access to the subway. Make a left upon exiting the station, and at the end of the street, go up the steps to your left to get on the boardwalk beside the tracks, which traverses one sinuous inlet of Jamaica Bay (walking through the streets would make the trip half again as long). Step off the subway shortcut at Russell St. and 104th St. The subway runs on a line constructed in the late 19th century for a railroad, which would make a stop here at Russell St.

- Proceed on 104th, the only north–south street. On your right three blocks along is the home of one of the few volunteer fire departments left in the city. It carries the name West Hamilton Beach because there was still an East Hamilton Beach when the department was established in 1928—but it was swallowed up by the development of Kennedy Airport after World War II, so now Hamilton Beach and

QUEENS' OTHER ISOLATED TOWNS IN THE BAY

East of Kennedy Airport, in the neighborhood of Rosedale, are two Jamaica Bay communities that are even smaller, more remote, and lesser known than Hamilton Beach. **Warnerville,** abutting Thurston Basin, consists of two roads separated by a rivulet of the bay. You find **Meadowmere** (*below*) behind Rockaway Blvd. storefronts—four streets on a tiny wedge of land protruding into Hook Creek. Neither community has more than 25 houses, some of them run-down or abandoned. Meadowmere and Warnerville weren't connected to city sewer service until 2010 and still don't appear on every map, but they are fun discoveries for the urban explorer. Warnerville even has a restaurant, the Bayhouse, with a waterside patio. Meadowmere's only commerce is a seasonal bait shop, unless you count the IHOP on Rockaway Blvd. If you cross water while walking around Meadowmere, you've gone into Nassau County. A cute footbridge off 1st St. displays the name

MEADOWMERE PARK, which is the town on the Nassau side.

Combine a visit to Meadowmere or Warnerville with Brookville Park just north. A pond flows the half-mile length of the park, narrow as a stream in places, wider with a shoreline in others. You can crisscross it by footbridge, enjoying the foliage and bird-watching. Brookville Park is off Brookville Blvd. north of 147th Ave.; on the south side are the Hook Creek Wildlife Sanctuary and Idlewild Park Preserve, 160 acres of salt marsh. There's a kayak and canoe launch at the south end of Huxley St.; deteriorating pilings stick out of Hook Creek there, remnants of a discontinued rail line to the Rockaways. The railroad also left behind a furrow through the marsh grasses, visible from Edgewood St. off 149th Ave. To reach any of these places, take the Q113 bus from the F train at Parsons Blvd.

West Hamilton Beach are interchangeable. Superstorm Sandy wrecked all the fire department's trucks, ambulances, and equipment, and its fleet was replenished by donations from around the country. Among the vehicles it received were a fire engine that a Pennsylvania unit had sent to the crash of Flight 93 on 9/11 and a truck that had been donated to a Mississippi volunteer fire department after Hurricane Katrina. Continue past the firehouse on 104th St.

● All the streets off 104th dead-end at the water after one block, but you should go down one of them—say, James Ct.—to get an even better feel for the unusual surroundings. Residences in Hamilton Beach began as shacks and bungalows and have been getting larger and sturdier over the years, and today you can find everything from rattletrap cottages to rather elegant houses. Some of these blocks weren't mapped—or paved—until fairly recently. Another 21st-century change in Hamilton Beach: finally getting incorporated into the city sewer system. It's more or less at sea level here, so flooding is a threat even without a hurricane of once-in-a-lifetime magnitude.

● Go to the end of 104th St., past 165th Ave., the highest numbered avenue in Queens. The small park here is federal property, part of the Gateway National Recreation Area, which encompasses 26,000 acres in Queens, Brooklyn, Staten Island, and New Jersey bordering Jamaica Bay and the Atlantic Ocean. Follow the path next to the train tracks, and go to the right on the small beach. Another path through the reeds will bring you to the playground. Then head back on 104th St.

● Turn left at the firehouse onto Davenport Ct. Cross the pedestrian bridge at the end. It spans Hawtree Basin and offers an "Are you sure this is New York City?" view.

● Make a left off the bridge onto 99th St. in Old Howard Beach. This section between 95th and 99th Sts. was developed earlier than "new Howard Beach" to the west, and still has homes dating to the 1920s and 1930s. Like many other streets in Queens, on 99th, you find older homes that have retained their classic appearances amid those that have undergone gaudy makeovers.

● Cross 165th Ave. and go left onto the beachside path around Frank M. Charles Memorial Park—not a city park but part of the Gateway National Recreation Area. Proceed past the tennis courts to the flagpole, which honors servicemen from Howard Beach who died in wars and includes a 9/11 plaque. From this spot in the 1890s, businessman William Howard had a 2,000-foot-long pier erected, upon which he developed a resort with a hotel, dining room, dancing pavilion, more than a dozen bungalows, and a perpendicular pier that connected to the railroad. Howard's Landing had its own power plant that generated electricity, which was not yet commonplace. The illuminated hotel, with its turreted corner towers, was an alluring nighttime sight from the trains chugging across the bay. And then it all went up in flames in 1907, in an off-season fire that engulfed nearby boats and, according to the *New York Times,* "lit up Jamaica Bay for miles."

Continue along the path past the flagpole, or walk in the same direction on the beach. After his hotel burned down, Howard developed this beach for swimming and opened it to the public. It was so popular, though, that it eventually was restricted to those who lived in Howard Estates, the residential development he launched around 1910. He also added several amenities that exist in today's park, including tennis courts and a waterside walkway. These tennis courts, incidentally, produced a top-ranked pro: 1970s champ Vitas Gerulaitis, who grew up in Howard Beach.

From the beach, your Jamaica Bay panorama encompasses Kennedy Airport and both the subway and vehicular bridges to Broad Channel. You can see why the train was so vulnerable in a storm like Sandy, which trashed everything from signals to tracks and knocked the line out of service for seven months. Nowhere else in the 230-mile system is the subway so exposed—or so distant between stations.

● At the west end of the park, return to 165th Ave. The dining and business establishments across Shellbank Basin are located on Cross Bay Blvd., a main commercial drag of south Queens and the demarcation between old and new Howard Beach, the latter generally developed after World War II.

Wait at 96th St. for the Elmhurst-bound Q11 bus to the A train's Howard Beach station, or stay on it longer to connect with the J, R, or M.

POINTS OF INTEREST

Hamilton Beach Park 104th St. and 165th Ave.

Frank M. Charles Memorial Park 99th St. and 165th Ave.

route summary

1. Take the boardwalk from the subway station to Russell St. and 104th St.
2. Walk south on 104th St.
3. Go in and out of James Ct.
4. Visit Hamilton Beach Park, then go back north on 104th St.
5. Turn left on Davenport Ct.
6. From the pedestrian bridge, turn left on 99th St.
7. Enter the park at 165th Ave.
8. Out of the park, get the Q11 bus on 165th Ave. near 96th St.

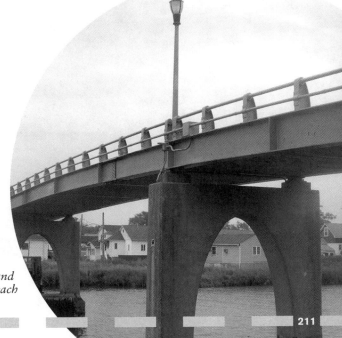

Pedestrian bridge linking Hamilton Beach and Howard Beach

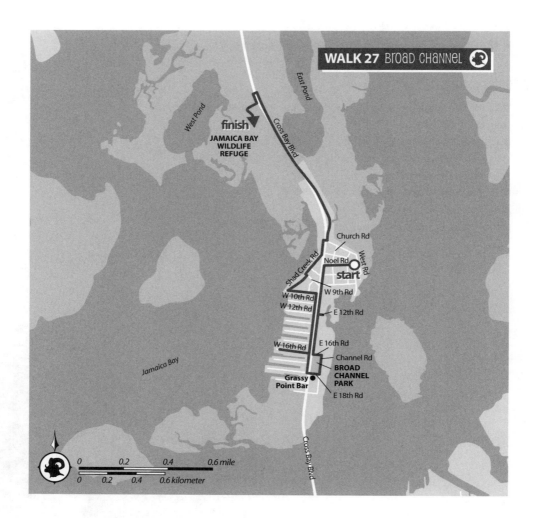

WALK 27 BROAD CHANNEL

East Pond

West Pond

Cross Bay Blvd

finish
**JAMAICA BAY
WILDLIFE
REFUGE**

Church Rd

Shad Creek Rd

Noel Rd

West Rd

start

W 10th Rd

W 9th Rd

W 12th Rd

E 12th Rd

W 16th Rd

E 16th Rd

Channel Rd

**BROAD
CHANNEL
PARK**

**Grassy
Point Bar**

E 18th Rd

Jamaica Bay

Cross Bay Blvd

0   0.2   0.4   0.6 mile

0   0.2   0.4   0.6 kilometer

27 Broad Channel: an Island That's Half for the Birds

BOUNDARIES: Jamaica Bay Visitor Center, West Rd., E. 18th Rd., Shad Creek Rd.
DISTANCE: 3 miles
SUBWAY: A to Broad Channel

New York City is an archipelago, and its better-known smaller islands—Liberty and Roosevelt, for example—are those dotted around Manhattan. The islands in Jamaica Bay, the estuary separating the Rockaway Peninsula from "mainland" Queens, are situated not only far from midtown but even fairly remotely from central Queens. Only one is inhabited by humans and accessible by any form of transport besides boat. Its real name is Big Egg Marsh, but it's called Broad Channel, the name of the residential community on the southern part of the island. No more than a quarter mile wide at most points, Broad Channel is one of New York's unlikeliest neighborhoods, where some homes are reached by footbridge, many have docks instead of backyards, and the commercial district comprises a few blocks of mom-and-pop businesses. North of the Broad Channel neighborhood, more than half the island is occupied by the Jamaica Bay Wildlife Refuge, another unlikely New York City locale. Upward of 325 bird species have been spotted in Jamaica Bay, and birding is a prime draw for the refuge.

● You arrive in the "Venice of New York" at NYC's most isolated subway station. The 3.5 miles from Howard Beach is the longest distance between stops in the entire 468-station subway system, and it's nearly 2 miles to the next stop in Rockaway. The A train was out of service here for seven months after Hurricane Sandy—it took three months just to clear all debris from the tracks. The storm mangled steel rails and destroyed part of the train's embankment. Post-Sandy, a new $16 million seawall for the Broad Channel section of the A line was designed to prevent any such future catastrophe. When you exit the station, walk on Noel Rd.

Two blocks along, Broad Channel's two churches stand on opposite sides of, no surprise, Church Rd. You first approach Christ Presbyterian By-the-Sea, which was so damaged by Sandy that it did not host services for 10 months. In typical Channel fashion, the rebuilding of the church was largely a community effort. The Catholic church St. Virgilius, Broad Channel's oldest religious congregation, dates to the first decade of the 20th century but now shares a priest with a parish in Rockaway. The firehouse across the street from the churches was erected soon after the volunteer fire department was established circa 1905, back when all of Broad Channel's houses were made of wood but the island was not served by the city's water supply or any vehicular bridges. Many local men still proudly and dutifully belong to the department, perhaps the most venerable institution in Broad Channel. This has traditionally been an insular community: If you know someone in Broad Channel, you probably know everyone. Families stay for generations, and residents are generally well versed in hometown history.

● Turn left on Cross Bay Blvd. The boulevard extends several miles north from the island, via the Congressman Joseph P. Addabbo Bridge, and runs south to Rockaway, but Broad Channel's other streets have no connection to the rest of Queens—and not just physically. Numbered roads preceded by *East* or *West* like you see off of Cross Bay Blvd. don't exist elsewhere in the borough and are not part of Queens' street grid.

At E. 9th Rd., Gene Gray Playground features a number of accouterments befitting this water-bound community, from the fish sculptures on the fence to the real anchor inside. You will probably notice other nautical-themed decor as you walk in Broad Channel—fish-shaped mailboxes at some houses, for example. The flamboyant corner building across the boulevard was one of several developments planned by a local entrepreneur intent on positioning Broad Channel as a vacation spot. It housed a drugstore with old-fashioned interiors but went out of business after just a few years. Broad Channel does have a history as a vacation destination: In the 1910s and 1920s, when it was a stop on the Long Island Rail Road (the tracks would be taken over by the subway in the 1950s), Broad Channel had hotels, bungalows, dance halls, and an outdoor cinema known as a "movie airdrome," which was located where today there's a commercial strip across from the playground.

● Proceed on Cross Bay Blvd. and make a left at E. 12th Rd. Steps from the major boulevard, you can see from here just how unusual Broad Channel is compared with other residential neighborhoods of New York: Marshes rather than roads separate rows of houses, and only wooden boardwalks (or boats) get people to the houses farther out in the bay—which are on stilts.

- Go back to Cross Bay Blvd. and continue south. Past E. 16th Rd., turn left into the park at the flagpole.

- Go straight through the park, and turn right onto Channel Rd., where some mini-mansions have been built. One reason Broad Channel's housing stock only recently began to expand and get more lavish is that until 1982 the city owned the land and residents just leased, but could not buy, their homes.

- Turn right on E. 18th Rd. On your left at Cross Bay Blvd. is the main local hangout, Grassy Point Bar. If you go in for a drink, be sure to see the display of historic Broad Channel photos in the rear; the bar is full of memorabilia and vintage kitsch. You're not far from the southern end of Broad Channel. From Grassy Point's front steps, you can see the tollbooths for the bridge to the Rockaways. But this walk takes you in the other direction.

- Turn right on Cross Bay Blvd. and check out the library on your right. Broad Channel didn't have its own branch until that 1980s change in land-ownership policy extended certain public services to the community. And then Channelites got a library that represents their heritage: It's shaped like a maritime rotunda.

- Turn left on W. 16th Rd. to see Broad Channel's unique streetscape: Canals separate the roads on the west side—they were created by reshaping the marshes for boat access. Return to Cross Bay Blvd. and make a left to continue heading north.

- Turn left at W. 10th Rd. and pass Power Rd., so named because it was the site of Broad Channel's original power plant. In those early days, the electricity didn't last 24 hours—a flashing light at the plant would let residents know to switch to gas for the evening. At the end of 10th, you'll have a terrific view of the Manhattan skyline and, to the left of it, the Verrazano-Narrows Bridge, a Doppler weather radar tower, and the Gil Hodges Marine Pkwy. Bridge, which connects Brooklyn and Rockaway.

- Walk on Shad Creek Rd. P.S. 47, on your right, is the rare NYC public school that includes both elementary and middle school grades—and it still has fewer than 300 students! (Kids go off-island for high school.) A number of the houses on the water side were modified and enlarged from the original 1920s and 1930s models; some of them were built for yacht clubs. All have arguably the finest view any New York City residence could offer.

- Make a left on W. 9th Rd. and a quick right to continue on Shad Creek Rd. Stay on it until you're back at Cross Bay Blvd., and turn left.

- Cross the boulevard to visit the small park honoring veterans on the median where the flagpole stands. Walk north along the local lanes. From where they merge into the main lanes of Cross Bay Blvd., it's less than a half mile north to the Jamaica Bay Wildlife Refuge. En route you'll pass the offices and "fleet" of Broad Channel's largest corporate citizen, Call-Ahead portable toilets. Past that, the water you see on your right is the biggest pond within the wildlife refuge.

- Proceed to the visitor center on your left to pick up a trail map and look at exhibits on the history, geography, and ecology of the area. The Jamaica Bay Wildlife Refuge is an important bird sanctuary and one of NYC's natural wonders—more than 9,000 acres of marshes, grasslands, channels, gardens, and ponds. In the midst of this nature, you'll have views of the subway train traversing the bay, arrivals and departures at JFK Airport, and the high-rise buildings in both Manhattan and Rockaway.

- After you've enjoyed the wildlife refuge, wait at a bus stop on Cross Bay Blvd. for the B53. You can take the bus south to Noel Rd., and walk back to the Broad Channel subway, or north and transfer to the A, J, or R train along the route.

POINTS OF INTEREST

Grassy Point Bar 18-02 Cross Bay Blvd., 718-474-1688

Jamaica Bay Wildlife Refuge nyharborparks.org/visit/jaba.html, Cross Bay Blvd., 718-318-4340

route summary

1. From the subway station, walk west on Noel Rd.
2. Turn left on Cross Bay Blvd.
3. Go in and out of E. 12th Rd.
4. Turn left into Broad Channel Park south of E. 16th Rd.
5. Turn right on Channel Rd.
6. Turn right on E. 18th Rd.
7. Turn right on Cross Bay Blvd.
8. Turn left on W. 16th Rd., but return to Cross Bay Blvd. and continue north.
9. Turn left on W. 10th Rd.
10. Head north on Shad Creek Rd. Make a left on W. 9th Rd. and then a quick right to continue on Shad Creek.
11. Turn left on Cross Bay Blvd.
12. Turn left into the Jamaica Bay Wildlife Refuge visitor center.
13. Exit the wildlife refuge onto Cross Bay Blvd. to get the bus.

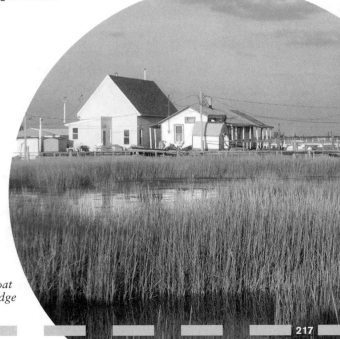

Broad Channel homes accessible by boat or footbridge

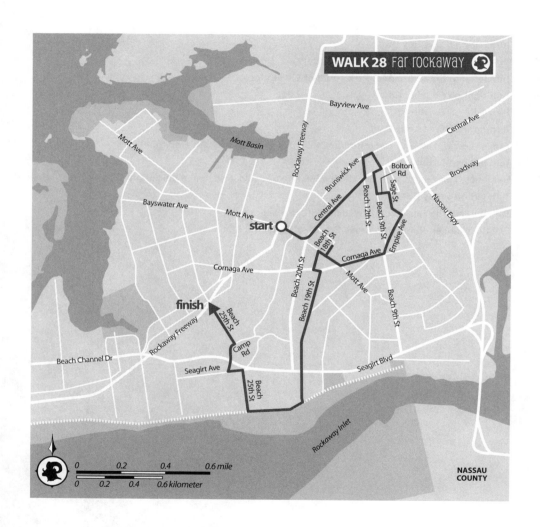

Bayview Ave

Central Ave

Mott Ave

Mott Basin

Rockaway Freeway

Brunswick Ave

Bolton Rd

Broadway

Mott Ave

Bayswater Ave

Mott Ave

start

Central Ave

Beach 12th St

Sage St

Beach 9th St

Empire Ave

Nassau Expy

Beach 18th St

Cornaga Ave

Cornaga Ave

Beach 20th St

Mott Ave

Beach 9th St

finish

Beach 19th St

Beach 25th St

Camp Rd

Rockaway Freeway

Beach Channel Dr

Seagirt Ave

Beach 25th St

Seagirt Blvd

Rockaway Inlet

0   0.2   0.4   0.6 mile

0   0.2   0.4   0.6 kilometer

NASSAU
COUNTY

28 Far rockaway: Beach Bungalow colony meets Business District

BOUNDARIES: **Brunswick Ave., Empire Ave., boardwalk, B 25th St.**
DISTANCE: **3.5 miles**
SUBWAY: **A to Far Rockaway–Mott Ave.**

There was a time when people couldn't wait to get to Far Rockaway, whether they were the well-to-do summering there around the late 1800s or, in later decades, working-class families who stayed in bungalows. Unfortunately, it's been a while since Far Rockaway was an alluring destination. Similar to Coney Island in Brooklyn, this once-fashionable resort that became a beach for all people suffered a terrible decline after World War II, with the construction of massive housing projects probably the most glaring culprit. But NYC's renaissance and an even more recent renewed appreciation of the Rockaways in particular have reversed the slide. Preserving the remaining bungalows has been one driving force in the ongoing renewal of Far Rockaway—which today is a typically Queens polyglot that includes people of African American, Jewish, Latino, and West Indian heritage. This is the largest, most urbanized, and most historic community on the Rockaway Peninsula.

Numbered streets throughout Rockaway are preceded by a B *for "Beach" or "Bay."*

● Several subway stations in the Rockaways have been enhanced with colored-glass artwork, and the vibrant seaside-inspired hues of artist Jason Rohlfe's *Respite* surround you as you leave the train. The bird theme is appropriate: The Rockaway Peninsula is bordered on the north by Jamaica Bay, home to hundreds of bird species, while stretches of its ocean beach (including one just west of Far Rockaway, starting around B 44th St.) are cordoned off every summer to protect nesting piping plovers. Out of the station, make a right on Mott Ave.

● Turn left on Central Ave. To your left, a splendid building more than a hundred years old features extensive terra-cotta ornamentation. Now a medical center, it was originally a bank, and the sight of it used to welcome Long Island Rail Road passengers

rockaway: The Lay of the Land

The 11-mile-long Rockaway Peninsula, referred to as either Rockaway or the Rockaways, is the westernmost link in a chain of barrier islands separating Long Island's south shore from the Atlantic Ocean. The Queens County line lies right where the peninsula branches off from the main body of Long Island. While some of Rockaway is directly south of Brooklyn, it all belongs to Queens. Its street numbering is separate from the rest of Queens. Vehicular access is via the Cross Bay Bridge in Queens, which enters Rockaway around Beach 94th St. or Brooklyn's Marine Pkwy. Bridge near Beach 169th.

Rockaway Park, Rockaway Beach, and Far Rockaway are probably the best-known neighborhoods, and the ones most visited by nonresidents. Other communities include Edgemere and Arverne toward the east; upscale Belle Harbor and posh Neponsit between the bridges; and the notoriously insular Breezy Point at the western tip (it's gated). Jacob Riis Park, which encompasses a full mile of beach-front and facilities like swings, basketball courts, picnic tables, and an Art Deco bathhouse, is part of the Gateway National Recreation Area, along with adjacent Fort Tilden, a decommissioned military complex with nature trails and beach areas. Rockaway had the longest boardwalk in the United States other than Atlantic City's prior to October 29, 2012, the date Hurricane Sandy pummeled the peninsula and destroyed the boardwalk west of Beach 88th St. It is not expected to be fully rebuilt until 2017.

to Far Rockaway. The adjacent strip mall went up where the train station had been before the LIRR relocated it a few blocks north in the 1950s. The older buildings and civic institutions nearby indicate the town center that developed around the station, but while the library and fire department are still here (on your right along Central), all that survives of the defunct local newspaper is its name on the Classical-style building across from the firehouse. The building with impressive brickwork at #15-18 has been vacated by the Masonic lodge that erected it in the late 19th century.

● Continue a few more blocks on Central, and you will reach First Presbyterian Church, also known as Russell Sage Memorial. It was designed by architects who worked on

Manhattan's St. John the Divine cathedral and contains a Tiffany window. Russell Sage was a politician, financier, and railroad tycoon whose wife, Olivia, inherited his entire fortune and spent it on philanthropy, including this 1910 church in the town where they used to have a summer home. The campuslike grounds, designed by the Olmsted Brothers (sons of Frederick Law Olmsted, the pioneering landscape architect most famous for Central Park), helped earn the church a spot on the National Register of Historic Places. Turn left on B 12th St., and then right on Brunswick Ave. and right on Sage St. to go around the whole property—and to see some old mansions neighboring it.

- Make a right from Sage St. back onto Central Ave. At B 9th St., check out the marker on the church lawn before going down that street, which evokes the era when people like the Sages lived in Far Rockaway. These large homes were often referred to as summer cottages then.

- Turn left on Bolton Rd. and then right on Sage St. The grand residences from a century ago give way to bland newer homes, and then the synagogue on your left after Balsam Ct. takes you back to the Space Age. Although Kneseth Israel has worshipped in this spaceship-shaped building since the mid-1960s, the synagogue is still commonly known as "the White Shul"—a nickname inspired by the congregation's former house of worship, a more Classical-style white building. The Orthodox Jewish population of Far Rockaway dwindled severely after the 1950s but has been surging since the 1990s and now dominates the western part of the neighborhood. Kneseth Israel is one of the original Orthodox congregations, established in 1922.

- Turn right on Empire Ave. The more elegant houses here are some of the priciest in Far Rockaway—and just a few blocks in the other direction on Empire is Nassau County's affluent "Five Towns." One of the Five Towns is Lawrence, and some call this area on the Queens side of the border West Lawrence.

- After Empire Ave. merges into B 9th St., make a right on Cornaga Ave. Cornaga meets Mott Ave. at Richard Feynman Way, named for the Nobel-winning physicist and Manhattan Project participant, who grew up in Far Rockaway.

- Go right on Mott Ave. In quick succession, you'll pass the police station and post office, both quite distinctive, as are the columned churches across from the post office. The post office was modeled after Thomas Jefferson's home, Monticello.

- Turn right on the street between the post office and the white church to see an unusual school design. Banks of skylights line this and another side of M.S. 53, also known as Brian Piccolo Middle School. Students voted on the school's name following the original airing in the early 1970s of the TV movie *Brian's Song,* which immortalized cancer-stricken NFL player Piccolo (who was portrayed by Queens-bred actor James Caan).

- Return to Mott Ave. to give that charming old country church, with its wooden bell tower and shingles, a good look. It was designed in the 1850s by Gothic master Richard Upjohn as a chapel of a Nassau County–based parish. The congregation eventually became independent, with the name St. John's Episcopal. Confused by what appears to be a Jewish name of the current occupant? Hyphens be damned, it's actually the Bethel Temple Church of God.

- Turn left from Mott Ave. onto B 19th St.

- Make a left on Cornaga Ave. and then a right to get back on B 19th. We are making our way to the beach through what used to be the Cornell estate. Richard Cornell, who ran an ironworks and was one of the wealthiest men in colonial New York, bought much of the land that's now Far Rockaway in the 1680s. His descendants were still parceling it up and selling it off well into the 1800s.

- Proceed south on B 19th St. The building at #264, after you cross Plainview Ave., recalls another aspect of Far Rockaway's history. Though it was the wealthy who first vacationed here, eventually there were accommodations catering to all classes. And the underprivileged were not excluded: Organizations that cared for poor, sick, or orphaned children had summer residences in Rockaway, and quite a few—including the Children's Haven of Far Rockaway, whose name is still on this building—were established here year-round. As you cross Seagirt Blvd., you're passing through the former grounds of the legendary Marine Pavilion. Cornell's home was demolished to make way for the opulent hotel, the first in the Rockaways and known throughout the country. The owners built a turnpike to Far Rockaway so guests could travel via stagecoach from Brooklyn and Jamaica. The hotel burned down in 1864; during its 30 years in operation, such luminaries as Henry Wadsworth Longfellow and Washington Irving signed the guest register.

- Take 19th right to the boardwalk.

- Make a right and walk west on the boardwalk for a short distance.

- Turn right on either B 24th or B 25th St., both blocks of true nostalgia. In the 1920s, bungalows were constructed en masse in the Rockaways, and for decades they provided a summer retreat for families of modest means. There were once about 7,000 of these homes; now just a few hundred remain, clustered in Rockaway Park and in this area known as Wavecrest.

- Turn left on Seagirt Ave. Make a right on Camp Rd. and a left on B 25th. Walk approximately a quarter mile to the A train's Beach 25th St. station.

route summary

1. Walk east on Mott Ave. from the subway station.
2. Turn left on Central Ave.
3. Go around First Presbyterian via a left on B 12th St., a right on Brunswick Ave., a right on Sage St., and a right onto Central Ave.
4. Turn left on B 9th St.
5. Turn left on Bolton Rd. and then right on Sage St.
6. Turn right on Empire Ave.
7. After Empire Ave. merges into B 9th St., make a right on Cornaga Ave.
8. Make a right on Mott Ave. and take a short side trip down B 18th St.
9. Turn left on B 19th St., left on Cornaga Ave., and then right on B 19th.
10. Make a right on the boardwalk.
11. Turn right on B 24th or 25th St.
12. Turn left on Seagirt Ave.
13. Make a right on Camp Rd.
14. Turn left on B 25th St. and proceed to the subway station on Rockaway Fwy.

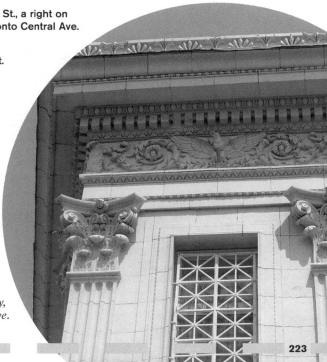

The former National Bank of Far Rockaway, on Central Ave.

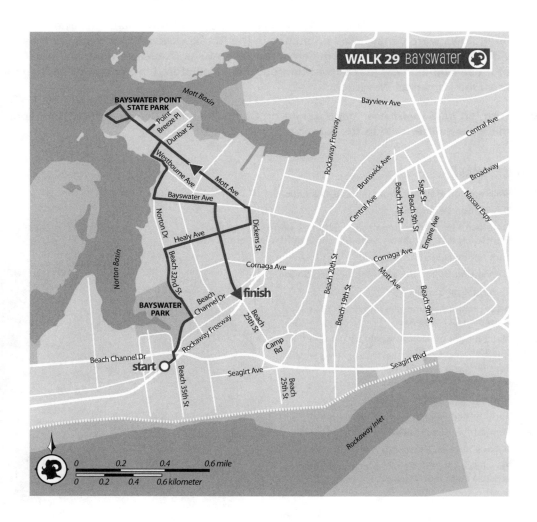

WALK 29 Bayswater

Mott Basin

BAYSWATER POINT
STATE PARK

Bayview Ave

Point
Breeze Pl

Dunbar St

Rockaway Freeway

Brunswick Ave

Central Ave

Broadway

Westbourne Ave

Mott Ave

Central Ave

Beach 12th St

Sage St

Beach 9th St

Empire Ave

Nassau Expy

Bayswater Ave

Dickens St

Norton Dr

Healy Ave

Cornaga Ave

Beach 20th St

Cornaga Ave

Mott Ave

Beach 9th St

Norton Basin

Beach 32nd St

Beach
Channel Dr

finish

Beach 19th St

BAYSWATER
PARK

Rockaway Freeway

Beach
25th St

Camp
Rd

Seagirt Blvd

Beach Channel Dr

start

Beach 35th St

Seagirt Ave

Beach
25th St

Rockaway Inlet

0   0.2   0.4   0.6 mile
0   0.2   0.4   0.6 kilometer

29 Bayswater: The Lost Resort

BOUNDARIES: Bayswater Point, Dickens St., Beach Channel Dr., B 36th St.
DISTANCE: 3.5 miles
SUBWAY: A to Beach 36th St.

Bayswater's identity is, of course, important to those who have lived here, but many outsiders do not know it as a place discrete from Far Rockaway. In the 1870s William Trist Bailey, a British-born mogul, created a community named Bayswater, where those of Bailey's social stratum would have their summer estates. Bayswater introduced foxhunting and yacht clubs to the Rockaways. Bailey built a hotel, but Bayswater was designed primarily for individual homes, and it stayed noncommercial while the Far Rockaway area began to fill with hotels and other businesses catering to vacationers. Eventually, as Rockaway opened up to the middle and working classes and as transportation improved and farther-flung locales were developed, Bayswater was usurped by destinations like the Hamptons. But it managed to elude the worst of the urban decay that overtook the Rockaways, and zoning laws kept out huge apartment complexes like those that went up in nearby Edgemere, Arverne, and Far Rockaway. The mansions that remain from Bayswater's heyday are not its only well-kept secret: There's also a state nature preserve.

Numbered streets throughout Rockaway are preceded by a B for "Beach" or "Bay."

- Use the northside exit from the subway station, and go down the stairs on your right. Walk straight ahead and turn left on B 35th St.

- Cross Beach Channel Dr., then go right to get onto Beach Channel Dr., walking with the grass and trees on your left. Marine-themed murals enliven Bayswater Park to your left. The water here is the Norton Basin, one of two basins bordering Bayswater, which occupies a nub of the Rockaway Peninsula jutting into Jamaica Bay.

- Turn left onto B 32nd St., or reach it by walking through the park. Continue past the ball fields, created for the Far Rockaway High School baseball team.

- Turn right on Healy Ave. The older houses of Bayswater date to the early 20th century, with some going back as far as 1900. You also pass two synagogues: Young Israel, past Hartman Ln., is an Orthodox congregation. The Bayswater Jewish Center, at Dickens St., is a Conservative synagogue that offers many social and cultural activities, including productions by the Bayswater Players, a community theater in existence for more than 50 years.

- Turn left on Dickens St.

- Turn left on Mott Ave. (Make sure you're on Mott rather than Bayswater Ave., which also branches off here in the same direction.) Some old houses may have been injudiciously modified or fallen into disrepair, but the avenue still sports enough porches, turrets, curved rooflines, and other classic elements to recall a bygone era.

  An interesting relic is on your right at Granada Pl.: pillars that say ELSTONE PARK, the name of a hotel and residential community developed here after Bailey's hotel, Bayswater House, went out of business. How much credit Bailey deserves for Bayswater is questionable, based on the surviving records. Some accounts say he developed an entire neighborhood, while others attribute only the hotel to him and say his plans for the area fizzled. And he may have been out of the picture before Bayswater flourished (Bayswater House shut down by 1905). It seems numerous lawsuits were brought against Bailey over debts and business deals, and he ended up in bankruptcy. His successors apparently didn't fare all that well with Elstone Park: There was a large-scale sell-off of properties as early as 1908, and while the hotel may have lasted into the 1920s, it went though many alterations.

- Turn right on Point Breeze Pl. On the left, Sunset Lodge's brick gateposts remain in finer condition than the circa-1910 house beyond them. The Audubon Society was bequeathed the home when its last owner died in the early 1980s, but the group ultimately turned over ownership to the state. Unoccupied for decades, it's now used by staff of the adjacent state park. Mainly, though, it stands as a local curiosity and reminder of vanished affluence. The house directly across the street, which is about a decade younger, is as nicely maintained as Sunset Lodge is neglected.

- Return to Mott Ave., make a right, and go to the end to visit the aforementioned state park, Bayswater Point. Follow the pebble path inside the gate, and when you reach a field, go right on the path that's been trod through the grass . . . all the way to the end of Bayswater, the shore of Mott Basin. This hideaway with an amazing Manhattan view is a favorite destination of fishermen—and birds. It's extremely peaceful, except for the roar of jets at nearby JFK Airport. From the concrete ruins of a pier, the residential area to your right is in Nassau County, and the nearest bridge to your left links Rockaway with the island community of Broad Channel.

- Walk with the water on your right to the ruins of another pier. Go onto the grass, pass picnic tables to your right, and wander on the lawn looking for remnants of a house's foundation. Built in 1907 by banker Louis Heinsheimer, the palatial estate was named Breezy Point, a name later taken by the neighborhood at the western end of Rockaway. The mansion was converted into a children's hospital in the 1920s but was unoccupied when it was ravaged by fire in the mid-1980s and subsequently demolished. The conservatory was left standing for a time, but now all that's left of it are these bits of tiled flooring.

- Watch on your left for a path between trees, and follow it back to Mott Ave.

- From Mott, make the first right after Point Breeze Pl., which is Dunbar St.

- Turn left at the water. This is Westbourne Ave. Stay to the right as you come around the bend so that you can continue walking along the bay. You'll be on Norton Dr.

- Turn left on Bayswater Ave. Pass Trist Pl., one of two Bayswater streets named for William Trist Bailey (Bailey Ct. is off of it).

- Make a right on B 25th St. At Cornaga Ave. is Far Rockaway High School, longtime pride of the neighborhood for its academics, athletics, school spirit, and this Collegiate Gothic building. The school graduated three future Nobel laureates (in physics and medicine), as well as pro-basketball player Nancy Lieberman, financier Carl Icahn, TV personalities Dr. Joyce Brothers and Richard Bey, and famous-for-the-wrong-reasons Bernie Madoff. Sadly, scholastic performance had deteriorated so severely that in 2011 FRHS was disbanded and reconstituted as a campus for several specialized public high schools, including ones focused on health careers, the arts and writing, and Spanish native speakers.

- Continue two blocks past the school to the Beach 25th St. stop for the A train.

POINTS OF INTEREST

Bayswater Park Beach Channel Dr. and B 32nd St.

Bayswater Point State Park Mott Ave. and Point Breeze Pl.

route summary

1.   From outside the train station, turn left on B 35th St.
2.   Make a right onto Beach Channel Dr.
3.   Turn left at B 32nd St.
4.   Make a right on Healy Ave.
5.   Turn left on Dickens St.
6.   Make a left on Mott Ave.
7.   Go in and out of Point Breeze Pl. on your right.
8.   Continue on Mott Ave. into Bayswater Point State Park.
9.   Head south on Mott Ave. after visiting the park.
10.   Turn right on Dunbar St.
11.   Go left on Westbourne Ave.
12.   Turn right on Norton Dr.
13.   Make a left on Bayswater Ave.
14.   Turn right on B 25th St.

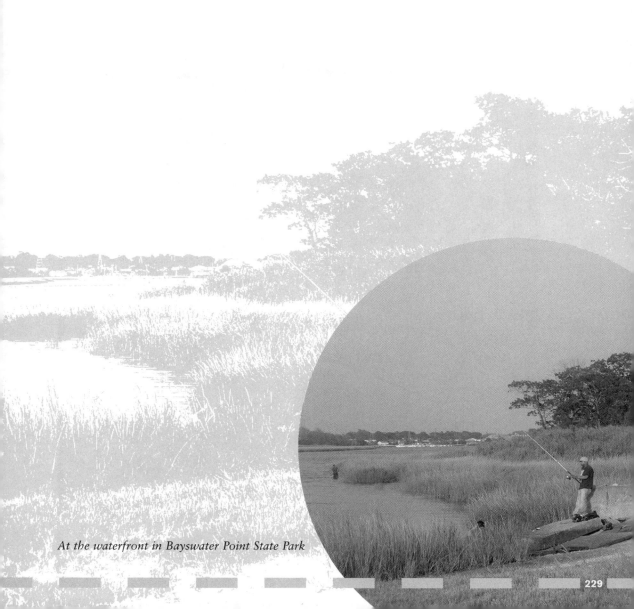

At the waterfront in Bayswater Point State Park

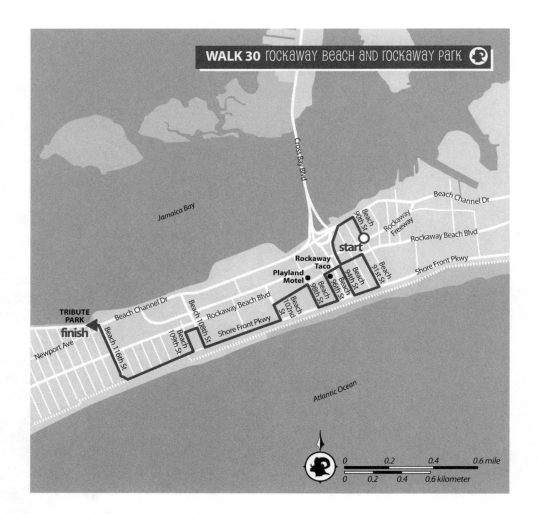

Cross Bay Blvd

Beach Channel Dr

Jamaica Bay

Beach 99th St

Rockaway Freeway

Rockaway Beach Blvd

Shore Front Pkwy

start

Rockaway Taco

Playland Motel

Beach 91st St

Beach 94th St

Beach 96th St

Beach 98th St

Beach 102nd St

Beach Channel Dr

Rockaway Beach Blvd

Shore Front Pkwy

Beach 108th St

TRIBUTE PARK

finish

Beach 109th St

Beach 116th St

Newport Ave

Atlantic Ocean

| 0 | 0.2 | 0.4 | 0.6 mile |
| 0 | 0.2 | 0.4 | 0.6 kilometer |

30 rockaway Beach and rockaway park: let the Good Times roll . . . again

BOUNDARIES: Beach Channel Dr., B 90th St., Atlantic Ocean, B 116th St.
DISTANCE: 3 miles
SUBWAY: A to Broad Channel, transfer to S to Beach 90th St.

Everyone's talking about Rockaway Beach's new hipster appeal, but weren't the Ramones singing about "Rock-Rock-Rockaway Beach" in the 1970s? Still, there's no doubt that Rockaway Beach has caught Williamsburg-itis of late, and while some are wary of the Brooklyn crowd, others give them credit for kick-starting a long-overdue renewal. Rockaway Beach and adjacent Rockaway Park were definitely on an upswing when Superstorm Sandy roared through in the fall of 2012 and destroyed their boardwalk; now, resurgence has a whole other meaning. A tour of these neighborhoods in the middle of the Rockaway Peninsula invariably covers a lot of what *used* to be there, and that's not just because of Sandy. The hotels, piers, and summer estates built during their first wave of development in the late 19th century are gone; so too are most of the bungalows that made them a working-class vacation paradise for much of the 20th century. This walk covers places of nostalgic and historic interest as well as some of the newer developments.

Numbered streets throughout Rockaway are preceded by a B *for "Beach" or "Bay."*

● Exit the train station via the stairs to your left on the north side of Rockaway Fwy. Make the first right, onto B 90th St. At the end of the block on the left, Rockaway's white elephant has stood vacant for more than three decades. Built in 1932, the courthouse was shut down when Queens County centralized its court system in 1962. After a brief life as a cultural center in the 1970s, the marble-and-limestone fortress has stayed empty, though it's due to be resuscitated as a medical center. A number of previous redevelopment plans, ranging from corporate offices to college campus, never came to fruition.

another part of the rockaways worth exploring

Take the Q22 or Q35 bus from Beach 116th St. to **Fort Tilden,** a decommissioned military installation built during World War I that's now under the auspices of the National Park Service. Enter the grounds at Rockaway Point Blvd. and Beach 169th St. A Nike missile stands on the grass as a reminder of the fort's last military function: Cold War anti-aircraft defense.

Walk west on Hann Rd. with the chapel on your left, passing a community garden and the buildings where the Rockaway Theatre Company performs and the Rockaway Artists Alliance mounts exhibitions and conducts classes.

Now that you've seen the area reclaimed by artists, move on to the part reclaimed by nature. Continue walking west, through a lot and onto the gravel trail in the so-called back fort, which has become maritime forestland (any DO NOT ENTER signs are meant for vehicles). Keep going

straight until you see a concrete edifice protruding from the foliage. This old gun battery has been outfitted with a staircase so that it can serve as an observation deck. Go up for an incredible panorama—from the ocean to the Verrazano-Narrows Bridge to the Manhattan skyline.

Back on the ground, take the sandy path opposite the battery, which will lead you down steps to Hidden Pond. From there, follow the trail through foliage to the beach. Its dunes, which reached as high as 25 feet, were virtually flattened by Superstorm Sandy, and the debris-strewn beach was closed for a year and a half.

Near the National Park Service signs farther east, a trail leads from the beach back to the fort. Across Rockaway Point Blvd., you can walk on the beach on the bay side, practically beneath the Gil Hodges Marine Pkwy. Bridge. In summer, ferries operate from Riis Landing there.

Fort Tilden's chapel, with the Marine Pkwy. Bridge beyond

- Turn left on Beach Channel Dr. Note the courts' names inscribed above their entrances. Continuing on Beach Channel Dr., you should see Jamaica Bay and the Cross Bay Veterans Memorial Bridge to your right.

- Cross B 92nd St. and go to your left on the street after it (next to the bridge access lanes). This is B 94th St., and you should follow it toward the First Congregational Church. Originating with Sunday-school classes in someone's home in 1881, the congregation dedicated its first sanctuary in 1888; this Georgian replacement dates to the early 1940s. Continue on B 94th St. across Rockaway Fwy.

- Turn left on Rockaway Beach Blvd., with the police station, firehouse, and library clustered on one block. The next couple of blocks feature some shops and eateries that have opened during Rockaway Beach's recent renaissance.

- Turn right on B 91st St. Cross Holland Ave., named for an influential family in Rockaway Beach's early history. Where you're walking was within the original 65 acres of farmland that the Hollands purchased in 1857 when they relocated from Jamaica; eventually, the whole area between today's 88th and 100th Sts. was known as Holland. The family ran an eponymous hotel and was involved in the founding of various civic institutions. On your left is a community garden that opened in 2011, transforming an abandoned lot into green space where residents can have their own plots. Art exhibits and other public events have been held here too.

- Turn right on Shore Front Pkwy. From 92nd down to 89th St., the beach is reserved for surfers; before that designation was made in 2005, surfing was illegal in New York City.

- Turn right on B 94th St.

- Make a left on Rockaway Beach Blvd., where there's an unusually gender-equitable tribute to veterans. The women's monument on the right was installed in the 1980s, joining the male statue dating to the 1920s. When the Doughboy was first erected, it stood like a sentry for Rockaway within a plaza right where cars came off the bridge; it was moved here when that earlier span was supplanted by a larger bridge.

- Turn left on B 96th St. Rockaway Taco, an indisputable factor in Rockaway Beach's revitalization, is on your left. A surfing restaurateur opened it in 2009 with a chef who'd worked in Mexico, and they've garnered particular praise for their fish tacos. Almost all ingredients are locally sourced—very local in some cases, as the restaurant owner has his own chicken coop and a rooftop farm. Rockaway Taco has spawned a culinary community, which includes its neighbors at this corner and some Brooklyn restaurants that have opened seasonal outlets at the boardwalk.

● Turn right on Shore Front Pkwy., then right on B 98th St. These condos have taken the place of Playland amusement park, the area's star attraction for generations. The fun house, bumper cars, and Atom Smasher roller coaster were probably the most popular rides. With a giant grinning clown face as its logo and the tagline "family fun since 1901," Playland put on a weekly fireworks show and hosted special events. The park outlasted most other tourist businesses in Rockaway Beach, as well as the Coney Island amusement parks that had been its rivals, and the end of an era was declared when park owners announced Playland would not reopen after the 1985 season. The name has been resurrected at Rockaway Beach Blvd., where the Playland Motel opened in 2013 in a 19th-century building refaced in distressed wood panels. The young, partying crowd that's rediscovered Rockaway immediately took to its bar, where the fun spills outside to a patio with beach chairs and, in an homage to the old Playland midway, games like cornhole and Ping-Pong. The hotel's guest rooms were each designed by a different artist according to a quirky theme.

● Walk west on Rockaway Beach Blvd., through the part of town that used to be called Seaside. It joined with Holland and the district to its east, Hammels, to form the village of Rockaway Beach in 1897, but when Queens County was merged into the City of New York a year later, its towns and villages lost their independence and became neighborhoods. St. Camillus, whose convent and church you pass on the left, started as a seasonal parish.

● Make a left on B 102nd St.

● Turn right on Shore Front Pkwy. to begin the oceanside segment of the walk—within the area where Superstorm Sandy ripped out the boardwalk. Walk on the beach if you wish.

● Turn right on B 108th St., where a bungalow colony has sprung back to life. Bunga-lows were the quintessential lodging of the Rockaways, and at least 7,000 of them existed on the peninsula at one time. Now only a couple of clusters are left, here and in Far Rockaway. Those in Far Rockaway front the streets, whereas these are situated along interior walkways.

● Turn left on Rockaway Beach Dr. and left on B 109th St. Past the playground, bungalow courts extend from both sides.

● At Shore Front Pkwy., go around the hockey rink and onto the beach to proceed west. You are now in Rockaway Park, a neighborhood that has its origins in a failed hotel venture. In 1880 the largest hotel in the world to date was constructed where you are walking. Bankers, railroad tycoons, and even senators invested in a 1,000-room hotel known as the Imperial, which consisted of a main building facing the ocean that stretched all the way from 109th to 116th St. and three wings extending north. It even had a private dock for guests arriving by steamer . . . except they never arrived. Mired in debt and lawsuits, the hotel never opened and was torn down in 1889 after standing empty for years. Wood and bricks from its demolition provided materials for early real estate development in the neighborhood. Meanwhile, the hotel was expunged from the résumé of its architect, Napoleon LeBrun, whose firm would design the world's tallest building in 1909, the Metropolitan Life Insurance tower on Madison Square Park in Manhattan.

● Leave the beach at 116th St. Colorful mosaics contrast with the somber monument across the walkway. The curved wall of granite blocks is a memorial to the 265 people killed when Flight 587 crashed in the Rockaways on November 12, 2001, minutes after taking off from Kennedy Airport. Five people on the ground perished along with all the passengers and crew on the Dominican Republic–bound flight. The disaster struck a community not only jittery from 9/11 but also still grieving the more than 55 residents who died at the Twin Towers. The quote above the arch comes from Dominican poet Pedro Mir and is inscribed in Spanish on the other side.

● Proceed up B 116th St. When Rockaway Park was developed around the turn of the century, retail establishments were confined to this street, and while the commercial district has expanded, it remains the main strip. Old buildings and businesses, including a shuttered 1920s movie theater and former flophouses, mix with newer entities as the three-block street continues to improve from its dodgiest days. The landmarked firehouse near the end on your left was built in 1913 with an open-air gallery at the top.

● Cross Newport Ave. and Beach Channel Dr. to enter Tribute Park, a beautifully designed 9/11 memorial with a view of lower Manhattan. In the center is a tile mosaic of a starburst encircled by the names of Rockaway neighborhoods. A separate monument dedicated to the firefighters features a ceramic replica of a helmet atop a boulder, and a twisted piece of steel from the World Trade Center wreckage is also on display. At the water's edge is a cupola designed by a local artist on which each glass star is imprinted with the name of a Rockaways resident who died in the attacks.

● B 116th St. has a subway station one block south of the park.

POINTS OF INTEREST

Rockaway Taco rockawaytaco.com, 95-19 Rockaway Beach Blvd., 347-213-7466
Playland Motel playlandmotel.com, 97-20 Rockaway Beach Blvd., 347-954-9063
Tribute Park rockawaytributepark.org, B 116th St. and Beach Channel Dr.

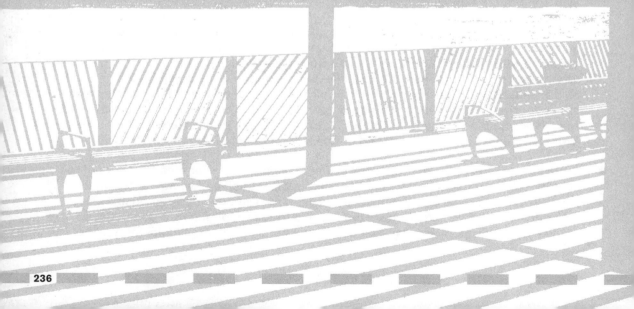

route summary

1. Walk north on B 90th St. from Rockaway Fwy.
2. Turn left on Beach Channel Dr.
3. Go left on B 94th St.
4. Turn left on Rockaway Beach Blvd.
5. Turn right on B 91st St.
6. Make a right on Shore Front Pkwy.
7. Turn right on B 94th St.
8. Make a left on Rockaway Beach Blvd.
9. Turn left on B 96th St.
10. Turn right on Shore Front Pkwy.
11. Make a right on B 98th St.
12. Make a left on Rockaway Beach Blvd.
13. Turn left on B 102nd St.
14. Turn right on Shore Front Pkwy.
15. Turn right on B 108th St.
16. Turn left on Rockaway Beach Dr.
17. Turn left on B 109th St.
18. Walk west on the beach.
19. Go right onto B 116th St.
20. After visiting Tribute Park, go south on B 116th St. to the subway.

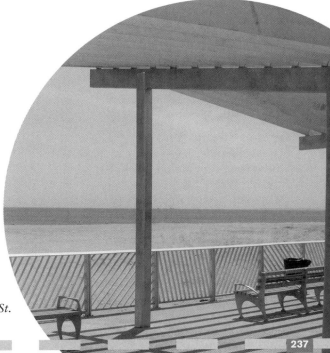

The beach near 106th St.

Appendix 1: WaLKS BY THeme

DINING, arts, and culture

Long Island City (Walk 1)
Astoria (South) (Walk 2)
Astoria (North) (Walk 3)
Sunnyside and Woodside (Walk 4)
Jackson Heights (Walk 5)
Flushing Meadows Corona Park (Walk 8)
Forest Hills (Walk 9)
Flushing (Walk 10)
Jamaica and Jamaica Hills (Walk 19)
Ridgewood (Walk 24)
Rockaway Beach and Rockaway Park
       (Walk 30)

residential Gems

Jackson Heights (Walk 5)
Forest Hills (Walk 9)
Whitestone and Malba (Walk 12)
Bayside (Walk 14)
Douglaston and Little Neck (Walk 15)
St. Albans (Walk 18)
Jamaica Estates (Walk 20)
Kew Gardens (Walk 21)
Richmond Hill (Walk 22)

ethnic Heritage

Astoria (South) (Walk 2)
Astoria (North) (Walk 3)
Sunnyside and Woodside (Walk 4)
Jackson Heights (Walk 5)
Elmhurst (Walk 6)
Corona (Walk 7)
Flushing (Walk 10)
Ridgewood (Walk 24)
Maspeth (Walk 25)

rich in History

Long Island City (Walk 1)
Astoria (South) (Walk 2)
Astoria (North) (Walk 3)
Elmhurst (Walk 6)
Flushing Meadows Corona Park (Walk 8)
Flushing (Walk 10)
Fort Totten to Beechhurst (Walk 13)
Jamaica and Jamaica Hills (Walk 19)
Woodhaven (Walk 23)
Ridgewood (Walk 24)
Far Rockaway (Walk 28)

Waterfront

Long Island City (Walk 1)
Astoria (North) (Walk 3)
College Point (Walk 11)
Whitestone and Malba (Walk 12)
Fort Totten to Beechhurst (Walk 13)
Bayside (Walk 14)
Douglaston and Little Neck (Walk 15)
Hamilton Beach and Howard Beach
(Walk 26)
Broad Channel (Walk 27)
Far Rockaway (Walk 28)
Bayswater (Walk 29)
Rockaway Beach and Rockaway Park
(Walk 30)

Pop-Culture Connections

Astoria (South) (Walk 2)
Corona (Walk 7)
Flushing Meadows Corona Park (Walk 8)
Forest Hills (Walk 9)
Fort Totten to Beechhurst (Walk 13)
Bayside (Walk 14)
Queens Village (Walk 17)
St. Albans (Walk 18)
Woodhaven (Walk 23)

Parks and Nature

Flushing Meadows Corona Park (Walk 8)
Bayside (Walk 14)
Alley Pond Park (Walk 16)
Kew Gardens (Walk 21)
Richmond Hill (Walk 22)
Woodhaven (Walk 23)
Broad Channel (Walk 27)
Bayswater (Walk 29)

Undiscovered or Farther Afield

College Point (Walk 11)
Whitestone and Malba (Walk 12)
Queens Village (Walk 17)
St. Albans (Walk 18)
Maspeth (Walk 25)
Hamilton Beach and Howard Beach
(Walk 26)
Bayswater (Walk 29)

Appendix 2: POINTS OF INTEREST

FOOD AND DRINK

Astor Bake Shop astor-bakeshop.com, 12-23 Astoria Blvd., Astoria, NY 11102, 718-606-8439 (Walk 3)

The Astor Room astorroom.com, 34-12 36th St., Astoria, NY 11106, 718-255-1947 (Walk 2)

Bareburger bareburger.com, 33-21 31st Ave., Astoria, NY 11106, 718-777-7011 (Walk 2)

Breadbox Café breadboxcafelic.com, 47-11 11th St., Long Island City, NY 11101, 718-389-9700 (Walk 1)

Cascarino's cascarinos.com, 152-59 10th Ave., Whitestone, NY 11357, 718-746-4370 (Walk 13)

Chao Thai 85-03 Whitney Ave., Elmhurst, NY 11373, 718-424-4999 (Walk 6)

Coffeed coffeednyc.com, 37-18 Northern Blvd., Long Island City, NY 11101, 718-606-1299 (Walk 2)

Corona Park Pork Store coronaparkporkstore.com, 150-54 14th Ave., Whitestone, NY 11357, 718-767-2654 (Walk 12)

Dani's House of Pizza danishouseofpizza.com, 81-28 Lefferts Blvd., Kew Gardens, NY 11415, 718-846-2849 (Walk 21)

Djerdan djerdan.com, 34-04 31st Ave., Astoria, NY 11106, 718-721-2694 (Walk 2)

Donovan's Pub donovansny.com, 57-24 Roosevelt Ave., Woodside, NY 11377, 718-429-9339 (Walk 4)

Empire Market empire-market.com, 14-26 College Point Blvd., College Point, NY 11356, 718-359-0209 (Walk 11)

Espresso 77 espresso77.com, 35-57 77th St., Jackson Heights, NY 11372, 718-424-1077 (Walk 5)

Freddy's Pizzeria 12-66 150th St., Whitestone, NY 11357, 718-767-4502 (Walk 12)

Glendale Bake Shop 69-25 Grand Ave., Maspeth, NY 11378, 718-457-2006 (Walk 25)

Grassy Point Bar 18-02 Cross Bay Blvd., Broad Channel, NY 11693, 718-474-1688 (Walk 27)

Himalaya Kitchen 86-08 Whitney Ave., Elmhurst, NY 11373, 718-213-3789 (Walk 6)

Hindu Temple Society of North America Canteen nyganeshtemple.org/canteen, 143-09 Holly Ave., Flushing, NY 11355, 718-460-8493 (Walk 10)

Iavarone Bros. ibfoods.com, 69-00 Grand Ave., Maspeth, NY 11378, 718-639-3623 (Walk 25)

Il Fornaio Bakery 29-14 30th Ave., Astoria, NY 11102, 718-267-0052 (Walk 3)

I Love Paraguay ilovepy.com, 43-16 Greenpoint Ave., Sunnyside, NY 11104, 718-786-5534 (Walk 4)

Jackson Diner jacksondiner.com, 37-47 74th St., Jackson Heights, NY 11372, 718-672-1232 (Walk 5)

Jamaican Flavors jamaicanflavors.com, 164-17B Jamaica Ave., Jamaica, NY 11432, 718-526-2228 (Walk 19)

Jollibee jollibeeusa.com, 62-29 Roosevelt Ave., Woodside, NY 11377, 718-426-4445 (Walk 4)

La Nueva Bakery lanuevabakery.com, 86-10 37th Ave., Jackson Heights, NY 11372, 718-507-2339 (Walk 5)

The Lemon Ice King of Corona thelemonicekingofcorona.com, 52-02 108th St., Corona, NY 11368, 718-699-5133 (Walk 7)

Leo's Latticini 46-02 104th St., Corona, NY 11368, 718-898-6069 (Walk 7)

Manducatis Rustica manducatisrustica.com, 46-35 Vernon Blvd., Long Island City, NY 11101, 718-937-1312 (Walk 1)

Manor Delicatessen manordeli.com, 94-12 Jamaica Ave., Woodhaven, NY 11421, 718-849-2836 (Walk 22)

Morscher's Pork Store morschersporkstore.com, 58-44 Catalpa Ave., Ridgewood, NY 11385, 718-821-1040 (Walk 24)

Nan Xiang 38-12 Prince St., Flushing, NY 11354, 718-321-3838 (Walk 10 addendum)

Neir's Tavern neirstavern.com, 87-48 78th St., Woodhaven, NY 11421, 718-296-0600 (Walk 23)

Nick's Pizza 108-26 Ascan Ave., Forest Hills, NY 11375, 718-263-1126 (Walk 9)

Norma's cafenormas.com, 59-02 Catalpa Ave., Ridgewood, NY 11385, 347-294-0185 (Walk 24)

Pates Plus patesplus.com, 97-15 Springfield Blvd., Queens Village, NY 11429, 718-468-9868 (Walk 17)

Playland Motel playlandmotel.com, 97-20 Rockaway Beach Blvd., Rockaway Beach, NY 11693, 347-954-9063 (Walk 30)

Premium Sweets 168-03 Hillside Ave., Jamaica, NY 11432, 718-739-6000 (Walk 19 addendum)

Rockaway Brewing Co. rockawaybrewco.com, 46-01 5th St., Long Island City, NY 11101 (Walk 1)

Rockaway Taco rockawaytaco.com, 95-19 Rockaway Beach Blvd., Rockaway Beach, NY 11693, 347-213-7466 (Walk 30)

Rudy's rudysbakeryandcafe.com, 905 Seneca Ave., Ridgewood, NY 11385, 718-821-5890 (Walk 24)

Sky Cafe 86-20 Whitney Ave., Elmhurst, NY 11373, 718-651-9759 (Walk 6)

Spicy & Tasty spicyandtasty.com, 39-07 Prince St., Flushing, NY 11354, 718-359-1601 (Walk 10 addendum)

Studio Square studiosquarenyc.com, 35-33 36th St., Astoria, NY 11106, 718-383-1001 (Walk 2)

Sweetleaf Coffee & Espresso Bar sweetleaflic.com, 10-93 Jackson Ave., Long Island City, NY 11101, 917-832-6726 (Walk 1)

Tortilleria Nixtamal tortillerianixtamal.com, 104-05 47th Ave., Corona, NY 11368, 718-699-2434 (Walk 7)

Performing arts

Astoria Performing Arts Center apacny.org, 30-44 Crescent St., Astoria, NY 11102, 718-706-5750 (Walk 3)

Black Spectrum Theatre blackspectrum.com, Roy Wilkins Park, St. Albans, NY 11434, 718-723-1800 (Walk 18)

Chain Theatre chain-theatre.org, 21-28 45th Rd., Long Island City, NY 11101, 646-580-6003 (Walk 1)

Chocolate Factory chocolatefactorytheater.org, 5-49 49th Ave., Long Island City, NY 11101, 718-482-7069

Illinois Jacquet Performance Space jazzatthechapel.org, 94-15 159th St., Jamaica, NY 11433 (Walk 19)

Jamaica Performing Arts Center jamaica-performingartscenter.org, 153-10 Jamaica Ave., Jamaica, NY 11432, 718-618-6170 (Walk 19)

Musica Reginae musicareginae.org, Church-in-the-Gardens, 50 Ascan Ave., Forest Hills, NY 11375, 718-894-2178 (Walk 9)

Oratorio Society of Queens queensoratorio.org, QPAC, 222-05 56th Ave., Bayside, NY 11364, 718-279-3006 (Walk 14 sidebar)

Queensborough Performing Arts Center qcc.cuny.ed/qpac, 222-05 56th Ave., Bayside, NY 11364, 718-631-6311 (Walk 14 sidebar)

Queens Symphony Orchestra queenssymphony.org, 65-30 Kissena Blvd., Flushing, NY 11367, 718-570-0909 (Walk 14 sidebar)

Queens Theatre queenstheatre.org, 14 United Nations Ave. S., Corona, NY 11368, 718-760-0064 (Walk 8)

Secret Theatre secrettheatre.com, 44-02 23rd St., Long Island City, NY 11101, 718-392-0722

Thalia Spanish Theatre thaliatheatre.org, 41-17 Greenpoint Ave., Sunnyside, NY 11104, 718-729-3880 (Walk 4)

VISUAL ARTS

Dorsky Gallery dorsky.org, 11-03 45th Ave., Long Island City, NY 11101, 718-937-6317 (Walk 1)

Dr. M. T. Geoffrey Yeh Art Gallery tinyurl.com/yehgallery, Sun Yat Sen Memorial Hall, St. John's University, Jamaica Estates, NY 11439, 718-990-7476 (Walk 20)

Fisher Landau Center for Art flcart.org, 38-27 30th St., Long Island City, NY 11101, 718-937-0727 (Walk 2)

Flux Factory fluxfactory.org, 39-31 29th St., Long Island City, NY 11101, 347-669-1406 (Walk 2)

Jeffrey Leder Gallery jeffreyledergallery.com, 21-37 45th Rd., Long Island City, NY 11101, 212-924-8944 (Walk 1)

MoMA PS1 ps1.org, 22-25 Jackson Ave., Long Island City, NY 11101, 718-784-2084 (Walk 1)

Noguchi Museum noguchi.org, 9-01 33rd Rd., Astoria, NY 11106, 718-204-7088 (Walk 3)

QCC Art Gallery qcc.cuny.edu/artgallery, 222-05 56th Ave., Bayside, NY 11364, 718-631-6396 (Walk 14 sidebar)

Queens Museum queensmuseum.org, New York City Building, Corona, NY 11368, 718-592-9700 (Walk 8)

Rockaway Artists Alliance rockawayartistsalliance.org, Studio 7 Gallery, Gateway National Recreation Area, Fort Tilden, NY 11695, 718-474-0861 (Walk 30 sidebar)

SculptureCenter sculpture-center.org, 44-19 Purves St., Long Island City, NY 11101, 718-361-1750 (Walk 1)

Socrates Sculpture Park socratessculpturepark.org, 32-01 Vernon Blvd., Astoria, NY 11106, 718-956-1819 (Walk 3)

Topaz Arts topazarts.org, 55-03 39th Ave., Woodside, NY 11377, 718-505-0440 (Walk 4)

HISTOrY

Bayside Historical Society baysidehistorical.org, 208 Totten Ave., Bayside, NY 11359, 718-352-1548 (Walk 13)

Bowne House bownehouse.org, 37-01 Bowne St., Flushing, NY 11354, 718-359-0528 (Walk 10)

Doughboy Plaza Woodside Ave. and 56th St., Woodside, NY 11377 (Walk 4)

Fort Totten Cross Island Pkwy. and Totten Rd., Bayside, NY 11359, 718-352-1769 (Walk 13)

Greater Astoria Historical Society astorialic.org, 35-20 Broadway, Astoria, NY 11106, 718-278-0700 (Walk 2)

King Manor kingmanor.org, 150-03 Jamaica Ave., Jamaica, NY 11432, 718-206-0545 (Walk 19)

Kingsland Homestead queenshistoricalsociety.org, 145-35 37th Ave., Flushing, NY 11354, 718-939-0647 (Walk 10)

Lewis H. Latimer House tinyurl.com/latimerhouse, 34-41 137th St., Flushing, NY 11354, 718-961-8585 (Walk 10)

Louis Armstrong House Museum louisarmstronghouse.org, 34-56 107th St.,
Corona, NY 11368, 718-478-8274 (Walk 7)

Maple Grove Cemetery maplegrove.biz, 127-15 Kew Gardens Rd., Kew Gardens, NY 11415,
718-544-3600 (Walk 21 sidebar)

Poppenhusen Institute poppenhuseninstitute.org, 114-04 14th Rd., College Point, NY 11356,
718-358-0067 (Walk 11)

Tribute Park rockawaytributepark.org, B 116th St. and Beach Channel Dr., Rockaway
Park, NY 11694 (Walk 30)

Vander Ende–Onderdonk House onderdonkhouse.org, 18-20 Flushing Ave.,
Ridgewood, NY 11385, 718-456-1776 (Walk 24)

Voelker Orth Museum vomuseum.org, 149-19 38th Ave., Flushing, NY 11354, 718-359-6227
(Walk 10 sidebar)

Parks

Alley Pond Park Cloverdale Blvd. and 46th Ave., Bayside, NY 11361 (Walk 16)

Astoria Park 19th St. and 23rd Terr., Astoria, NY 11105 (Walk 3)

Athens Square 30th Ave. and 29th St., Astoria, NY 11102 (Walk 3)

Baisley Pond Park Sutphin Blvd. and Rockaway Blvd., Jamaica, NY 11434 (Walk 19 sidebar)

Bayswater Park Beach Channel Dr. and B 32nd St., Far Rockaway, NY 11691 (Walk 29)

Bayswater Point State Park Mott Ave. and Point Breeze Pl., Far Rockaway, NY 11691
(Walk 29)

Brookville Park Brookville Blvd. and 147th Ave., Rosedale, NY 11422 (Walk 26 sidebar)

Captain Tilly Park Highland Ave. and 165th St., Jamaica Hills, NY 11432 (Walk 19 addendum)

Crocheron Park 35th Ave. and 216th St., Bayside, NY 11361 (Walk 14)

Dutch Kills Green Queens Plaza N. and 41st Ave., Long Island City, NY 11101 (Walk 2)

Elmhurst Park Grand Ave. and 79th St., Elmhurst, NY 11373 (Walk 25)

Flushing Meadows Corona Park Roosevelt Ave. and 114th St., Corona, NY 11368 (Walk 8)

Forest Park Park Ln. S. and Metropolitan Ave., Kew Gardens, NY 11415 (Walks 21, 22, and 23)

Francis Lewis Park 3rd Ave. and 147th St., Whitestone, NY 11357 (Walk 12)

Frank M. Charles Memorial Park 99th St. and 165th Ave., Howard Beach, NY 11414 (Walk 26)

Frontera Park Brown Pl. and 58th Ave., Maspeth, NY 11378 (Walk 25)

Gantry Plaza State Park Center Blvd. and 49th Ave., Long Island City, NY 11101, 718-786-6385 (Walk 1)

Hamilton Beach Park 104th St. and 165th Ave., Howard Beach, NY 11414 (Walk 26)

Hermon A. MacNeil Park Poppenhusen Ave. and 115th St., College Point, NY 11356 (Walk 11)

Hunters Point South Park Center Blvd. and Borden Ave., Long Island City, NY 11101 (Walk 1)

John Golden Park 33rd Ave. and 215th Pl., Bayside, NY 11361 (Walk 14)

Lance Corporal Thomas P. Noonan Jr. Playground Greenpoint Ave. and 42nd St., Sunnyside, NY 11104 (Walk 4)

Little Bay Park Cross Island Pkwy. between Utopia Pkwy. and Totten Rd., Bayside, NY 11360 (Walk 13)

MacDonald Park Queens Blvd. and 70th Ave., Forest Hills, NY 11375 (Walk 9)

Moore Homestead Playground Broadway and 45th Ave., Elmhurst, NY 11373 (Walk 6)

Park of the Americas 104th St. and 42nd Ave., Corona, NY 11368 (Walk 7)

Queens Village Veterans Plaza Jamaica Ave. and Springfield Blvd., Queens Village, NY 11428 (Walk 17)

Roy Wilkins Park Baisley Blvd. and Merrick Blvd., St. Albans, NY 11434 (Walk 18)

Rufus King Park 90th Ave. and 150th St., Jamaica, NY 11432 (Walk 19)

St. Albans Park Merrick Blvd. and Sayres Ave., Jamaica, NY 11433 (Walk 18)

Travers Park 34th Ave. and 77th St., Jackson Heights, NY 11372 (Walk 5)

Wayanda Park Hollis Ave. and Robard Ln., Queens Village, NY 11429 (Walk 17)

Windmuller Park Woodside Ave. and 54th St., Woodside, NY 11377 (Walk 4)

eDUCaTIONaL aND CULTUraL INSTITUTIONS

Central Library queenslibrary.org/central-library, 89-11 Merrick Blvd., Jamaica, NY 11432, 718-990-0700 (Walk 19 addendum)

Ch'an Meditation Center chancenter.org, 90-56 Corona Ave., Elmhurst, NY 11373, 718-592-6593 (Walk 6)

Flushing Town Hall flushingtownhall.org, 137-35 Northern Blvd., Flushing, NY 11354, 718-463-7700 (Walk 10)

Gottscheer Hall gottscheerhall.com, 657 Fairview Ave., Ridgewood, NY 11385, 718-366-3030 (Walk 24)

Jamaica Center for Arts & Learning jcal.org, 161-04 Jamaica Ave., Jamaica, NY 11432, 718-658-7400 (Walk 19)

Kupferberg Holocaust Resource Center and Archives qcc.cuny.edu/khrca, 222-05 56th Ave., Bayside, NY 11364, 718-281-5770 (Walk 14 sidebar)

Langston Hughes Community Library and Cultural Center queenslibrary.org/branch /langston-hughes, 100-01 Northern Blvd., Corona, NY 11368, 718-651-1100 (Walk 7)

Maria Rose International Doll Museum & Cultural Center mariarose.biz, 187-11 Linden Blvd., St. Albans, NY 11412, 917-817-8653 (Walk 18)

Museum of the Moving Image movingimage.us, 36-01 35th Ave., Astoria, NY 11106, 718-777-6888 (Walk 2)

New York Hall of Science nysci.org, 47-01 111th St., Corona, NY 11368, 718-699-0005 (Walk 8)

The Oracle Club theoracleclub.com, 10-41 47th Ave., Long Island City, NY 11101, 917-519-2594 (Walk 1)

Queensborough Community College qcc.cuny.edu, 222-05 56th Ave., Bayside, NY 11364, 718-631-6262 (Walk 14 sidebar)

Queens College qc.cuny.edu, 65-30 Kissena Blvd., Flushing, NY 11367, 718-997-5000 (Walk 14 sidebar)

Reso Box resobox.com, 41-26 27th St., Long Island City, NY 11101, 718-784-3680 (Walk 2)

Steinway & Sons steinway.com, 1 Steinway Pl., Astoria, NY 11105, 718-721-2600 (Walk 3 sidebar)

St. John's University stjohns.edu, 8000 Utopia Pkwy., Jamaica Estates, NY 11439, 718-990-2000 (Walk 20)

York College york.cuny.edu, 94-20 Guy R. Brewer Blvd., Jamaica, NY 11451, 718-262-2000 (Walk 19)

Sports and Recreation

Bayside Marina baysidemarinany.com, Cross Island Pkwy. and 28th Ave., Bayside, NY 11360, 718-229-0097 (Walk 14)

Citi Field tinyurl.com/citifieldnyc, Roosevelt Ave. and 126th St., Flushing, NY 11368, 718-507-8499 (Walk 8)

Forest Park Carousel forestparkcarousel.com, Woodhaven Blvd. and Forest Park Dr., Woodhaven, NY 11421 (Walk 23)

Idlewild Park Preserve Canoe and Kayak Launch Huxley St. and Craft Ave., Rosedale, NY 11422 (Walk 26 sidebar)

Joe Michaels Mile Cross Island Pkwy. between Northern Blvd. and Totten Rd., Bayside, NY 11360 (Walk 14)

LIC Community Boathouse licboathouse.org, 5th St. and N. Basin Rd., Long Island City, NY 11101 (Walk 1)

London Planetree Playground Atlantic Ave. and 88th St., Ozone Park, NY 11416 (Walk 23)

USTA Billie Jean King National Tennis Center tinyurl.com/bjktennis, Flushing Meadows Corona Park, Corona, NY 11368, 718-760-6200 (Walk 8)

World's Fair Marina and Flushing Bay Promenade Grand Central Pkwy. and 31st Dr., Corona, NY 11368 (Walk 7 addendum)

Flora and Fauna

Alley Pond Environmental Center alleypond.com, 228-06 Northern Blvd., Douglaston, NY 11362, 718-229-4000 (Walk 16)

Aurora Pond Udall's Cove Park, Bayshore Blvd. and Douglas Rd., Little Neck, NY 11363 (Walk 15)

Brooklyn Grange brooklyngrangefarm.com, 37-18 Northern Blvd., Long Island City, NY 11101, 347-670-3660 (Walk 2)

Evergreen Community Garden Colden St. at Juniper Ave., Flushing, NY 11355 (Walk 10 addendum)

Fort Tilden nyharborparks.org/visit/foti.html, Gateway National Recreation Area, Rockaway Point Blvd., Fort Tilden, NY 11695, 718-318-4300 (Walk 30 sidebar)

Jamaica Bay Wildlife Refuge nyharborparks.org/visit/jaba.html, Gateway National Recreation Area, Cross Bay Blvd., Broad Channel, NY 11693, 718-318-4340 (Walk 27)

Queens Botanical Garden queensbotanical.org, 43-50 Main St., Flushing, NY 11355, 718-886-3800 (Walk 10 addendum)

Queens County Farm Museum queensfarm.org, 73-50 Little Neck Pkwy., Floral Park, NY 11004, 718-347-3276 (Walk 17 sidebar)

Queens Zoo queenszoo.com, 53-51 111th St., Corona, NY 11368, 718-271-1500 (Walk 8)

Udall's Wildlife Preserve Douglas Rd. and Richmond Rd., Douglaston, NY 11363 (Walk 15)

SHOPPING

Astoria Bookshop astoriabookshop.com, 31-29 31st St., Astoria, NY 11106, 718-278-2665 (Walk 2)

LIC Flea & Food licflea.com, 5-25 46th Ave., Long Island City, NY 11101, 718-866-8089 (Walk 1)

Queens Center shopqueenscenter.org, 90-15 Queens Blvd., Elmhurst, NY 11373, 718-592-3900 (Walk 6)

Ridgewood Market ridgewoodmarket.com, 657 Fairview Ave., Ridgewood, NY 11385, 347-460-7549 (Walk 24)

INDEX

MAR – – 2016

about the author

ADRIENNE ONOFRI is a native New Yorker who's lived in Queens for the past 25 years. Her previous book, *Walking Brooklyn: 30 Tours Exploring Historical Legacies, Neighborhood Culture, Side Streets, and Waterways,* helped launch Wilderness Press's urban-trekking series. A licensed NYC sightseeing guide, Adrienne has led tours in Queens, Brooklyn, and Manhattan by foot, bus, car, and trolley. She has been a staff editor at several travel-industry publications and is currently a freelance editor for national consumer magazines. She is also a theater writer and member of the Drama Desk.

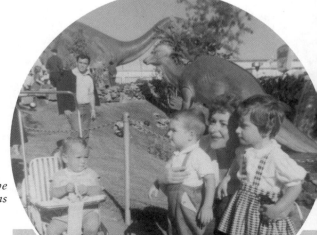

Adrienne (left) with her family at the 1964 World's Fair in Queens